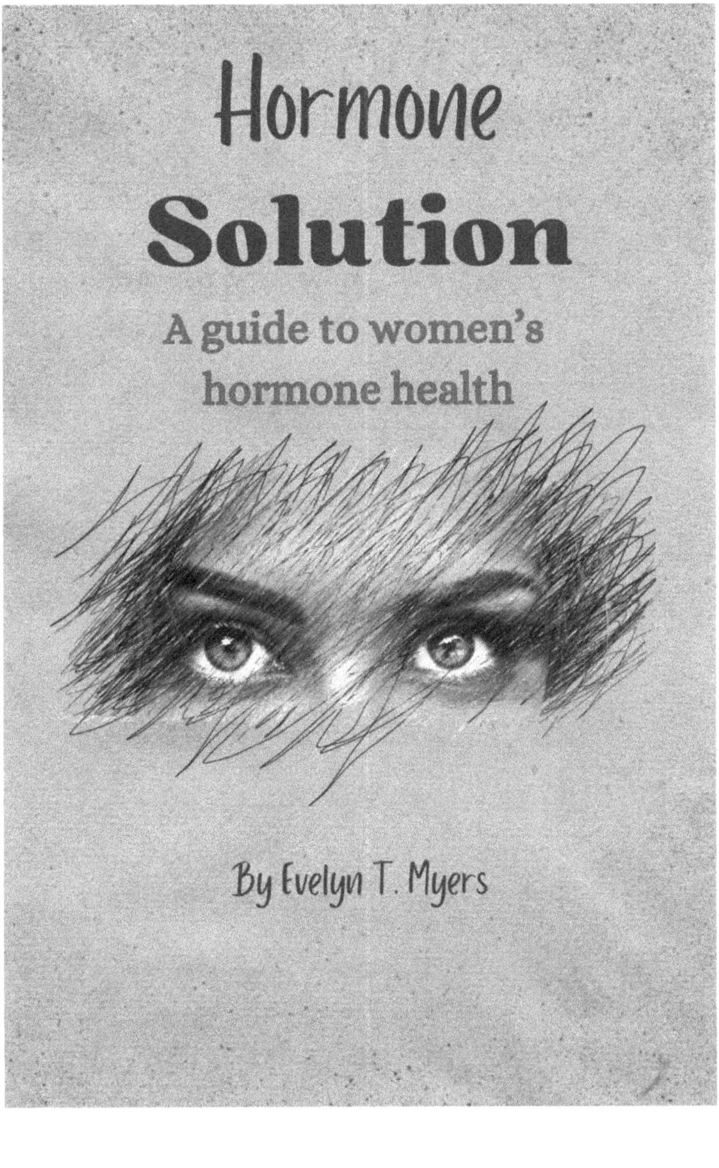

Hormone
Solution

A guide to women's hormone health

By Evelyn T. Myers

Hormone solution

A guide to women's Hormone health

Evelyn T. Myers

Disclaimer

The author of this book does not provide medical advise or prescribe the use of any technique as a form of treatment for physical, emotional, or medical problems without the direct or indirect counsel of a physician. The author's intention is just to provide broad information to assist you in your journey for emotional, physical, and spiritual well-being. If you use any of the information in this book for personal purposes, the author and publisher accept no responsibility for your actions.

TABLE OF CONTENT

	5
Introduction	**6**
Chapter 1	**17**
Perimenopause and menopause	17
Chapter 2	**39**
Embarrassment, Liberation, Sadness, and all in between	39
Chapter 3	**55**
The Importance Of Natural, Ovulatory Menstrual Cycles	55
Chapter 4	**67**
Second puberty's hormonal and physiological changes	67
Chapter 5	**109**
Perimenopause and beyond: general maintenance	109
Chapter 6	**171**
MHT (menopausal hormone treatment)	

171

Chapter 7   **197**

Difficulties with the body, including
allergies, thyroid illness, weight gain, and
aches and pains   197

Chapter 8   **254**

Estrogen : Crazy heavy periods and
breast pain   255

A FINAL WORD   **323**

Introduction

Welcome to Hormone Solution, your resource for healthy hormones after the age of 40.

If you've read my previous books, The Midlife Diet for Women and The Menopause Solution, you'll understand how passionate I am about women's hormones and health. In fact, you might say I'm an advocate for women's hormones and all the benefits that come with maintaining a healthy lifestyle.

With this book, I'm equally passionate about the final few years of perimenopause and the years following menopause. I didn't include the words perimenopause or menopause in the title because I didn't want you to think, 'Oh, this book doesn't apply to me,' when it very much does if you're 40 (or even near to 40).

Why am I so interested in perimenopause and menopause?
First and foremost, because it is happening to me. I'm 50 years old at the time of writing, and I've started

having long periods and forgetting where I parked my car. I'm also experiencing a new sense of cheeky independence, something I'd heard about from patients but hadn't fully grasped until it happened to me.

The second reason I'm interested in perimenopause and menopause is that I want to show how normal and typical it is. I'm doing so in reaction to an unofficial poll I ran on my social media platforms in which I asked, 'Are you terrified of menopause?' and 64% of women said yes. They stated being afraid of symptoms in the comments, which is understandable, but also being afraid of the stigma of menopause, which is also understandable but sad. How can society still stigmatize a basic natural process that affects 51% of the population?

We'll talk about stigma, and I'll try to offer some new perspectives on the subject. I'll also invite you to think of menopause as a distinct process from ageing, which is correct since, while perimenopause occurs alongside ageing, it's actually a separate process that is more analogous to second puberty. We'll look at the concept of second puberty and I'll argue that, from an evolutionary standpoint, menopause may have evolved as a favorable adaptation to allow for a longer human lifetime. Viewing menopause as a helpful adaptation is only one of various approaches to finding meaning in the process and moving beyond the commonly held belief that menopause is just the result of living too long.

How to Make Use of This Book

The first few chapters are all about comprehending the perimenopause process, both emotionally and physically, and include a discussion of the significance of regular ovulation. If learning about ovulation just as you're about to stop ovulating forever seems unusual, realize that's stopping ovulation' is the cause of the majority of symptoms that may emerge. To understand symptoms and how to manage them, you must first comprehend ovulation.

The book's final chapters are primarily about treatment. I'll present dietary and hormonal treatment techniques for symptoms ranging from heavy periods to weight gain to anxiety and night sweats, based on the most recent research and my own twenty-five years of dealing with patients. We'll start with a general maintenance chapter about the nervous system and diet, then move on to a detailed discussion of hormone therapy before going over each symptom separately and how to treat them with both conventional and alternative treatments. This book covers both the perimenopause process and the menopause life phase, which could last for more than four decades in total.

What essential new chapter in your life do you need to comprehend?

First, be aware that symptoms (if you encounter them) are probably only going to last a short time. Many perimenopausal symptoms are transient, though not all of them. Next, know that perimenopause is not merely an erratic "hormonal fluctuation," but rather a series of occurrences that start with low progesterone and temporary high estrogen levels and end with low estrogen and some important adjustments to insulin metabolism. Finding the best treatment will be made easier if you view the process as a series of observable occurrences.

Finally, be aware that even if you don't have any symptoms, perimenopause and the early years of menopause are a crucial time for your health. By "critical window," I mean a vulnerable moment or turning point during which minor health issues might, if not handled, worsen and become more severe later in life. An inflection point is advantageous because it provides a window of time for you to implement tiny changes that could have a significant positive impact on your long-term health.

Second puberty, or perimenopause, is a transient condition.

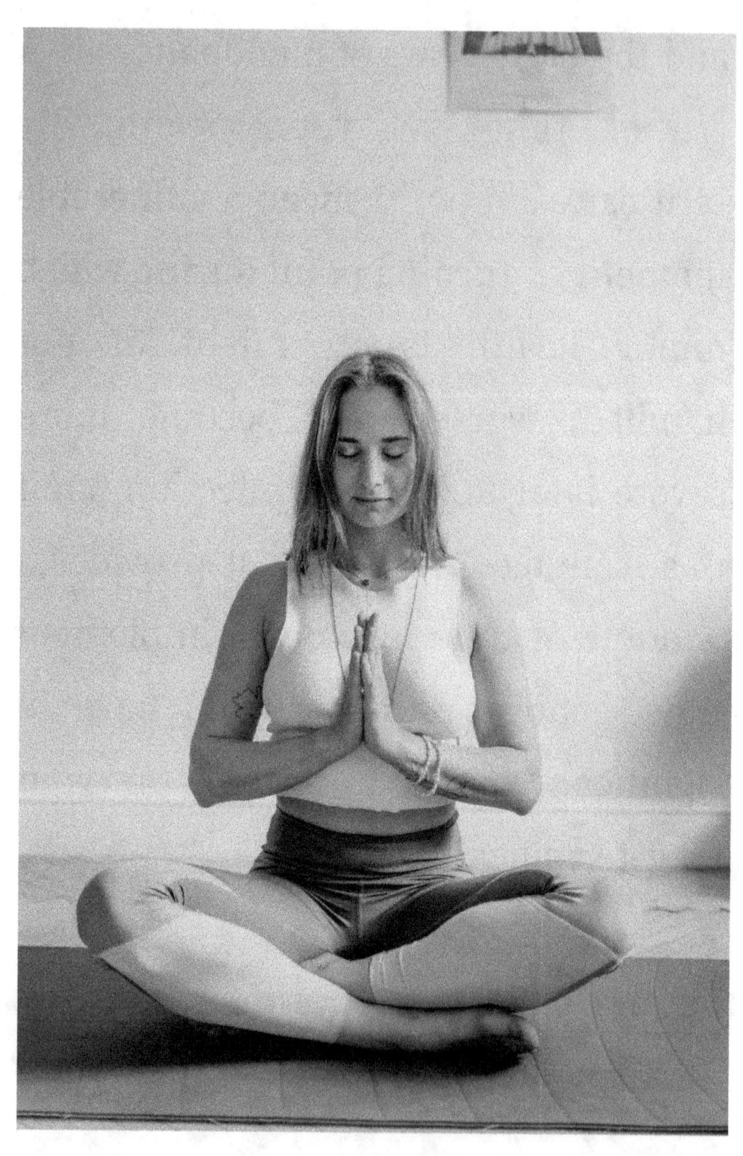

Chapter 1

Perimenopause and menopause

Something is changing with your body and, more specifically, your brain by your late thirties or early forties, and it can seem perplexing, irritating, and freeing all at the same time. The transition is not a single event, but rather a process known as perimenopause, which occurs two to twelve years before your periods stop.

Menopause, which begins one year following your last period, is not the same as perimenopause.

This book is about both the perimenopause process and the life phase of menopause, which can last for more than four decades.

What do you need to know about this significant new chapter in your life?

To begin, recognize that symptoms (if you encounter them) are likely to be transient. Not all perimenopausal symptoms are transient, but many are, and knowing this will keep you from thinking, "Oh, my goodness, this is how I'm always going to be now." This is not how you will always be; this too shall pass.

Next, recognize that perimenopause is not merely a chaotic 'hormonal fluctuation,' but a series of events that begins with low progesterone and ends with low estrogen and some major changes in insulin metabolism. Perceiving the process as a series of definable events will assist you in determining the best remedy.

Finally, understand that perimenopause and the early years of menopause are essential health windows, even if you don't experience symptoms. By the crucial window, I mean a sensitive period or inflection point at which time tiny health concerns may amplify into larger and more lasting health problems later in life if not handled. An inflection point also provides you with a window of opportunity to make tiny changes that could pay significant returns for your future health.

So there you have it: many symptoms are transient.

Perimenopause is the result of a series of events.

Perimenopause and the first few years of menopause are key health windows.

Age has nothing to do with perimenopause. You're obviously still young if you're 35 or even younger. Additionally, even if you are 50 years old, perimenopause occurs concurrently with aging but is unrelated to it.

The hormonal events and changes that occur during perimenopause are more analogous to those of puberty or second puberty. Especially in contrast to progesterone, the "period-lightening hormone," which is low until regular cycles are established, estrogen is high and fluctuating during the teen years. Both the first and second phases of puberty are characterized by high estrogen levels and low progesterone levels, with progesterone gradually increasing during the first phase and decreasing during the second. You may have had heavy periods as a teenager, and you may still have them in your forties due to high estrogen and low progesterone levels. You will eventually lose estrogen with second puberty and reach the comparable steady low estrogen of menopause. Symptoms may last ten years, but they won't last indefinitely because the hormone shift process may take ten years to complete. Therefore, you should think twice before adopting any diagnosis, such as fibromyalgia or chronic fatigue, as being unchangeable.

FIBROMYALGIA

Fibromyalgia is a disorder characterized by undiagnosed, persistent, widespread pain and a sensitive pain threshold. Women between the ages of 40 and 60 are commonly affected.

Heavy periods, pelvic pain, aching breasts, migraines, night sweats, and—most significantly—anxiety and sadness are additional transient symptoms of second puberty. Most studies indicate that the risk of anxiety and sadness increases throughout the perimenopause and then immediately decreases during menopause. Not all symptoms you experience in your forties are caused by perimenopause. Not at all. Consult your doctor if you have symptoms like pain or weariness as these could be signs of a more serious health issue. In addition to existing independently of perimenopause, thyroid disease can also be exacerbated or made worse by it. Because of how similar the symptoms are, it might even be mistaken for perimenopause.

The perimenopause is a series of occurrences.

Progesterone loss is the first step. Despite still having regular periods, you will begin to produce less progesterone sometime in your forties or perhaps late thirties.

Anxiety, breast soreness, heart palpitations, night sweats, recurrent headaches, and a myriad of other symptoms are just a few of the many things it can cause. Because perimenopausal symptoms are caused mostly by a decrease in progesterone rather than estrogen, progesterone, rather than estrogen, may be a preferable therapy option.

As your progesterone levels drop, you may begin to experience higher estrogen levels than ever before; in fact, up to three times higher, which can produce symptoms such as irritability, breast soreness, and heavy periods. High estrogen symptoms are caused by both the hormone's direct actions and the hormone's indirect effects on mast cells and histamine. Perimenopausal hot flushes are caused by an increase in estrogen and a drop from high to low levels, which implies that flushes while you're still having periods are more likely to be caused by progesterone rather than estrogen.

After your final period, you'll enter the zone of lower estrogen, which is simply that: lower estrogen, not deficient estrogen, because there's nothing 'deficient' about having the normal level of hormone for the life phase you're in. Also, as we'll see, you still produce a reasonable quantity of estrogen during that time, but it fluctuates, so many of the symptoms are caused by the dip from high to low. Menopausal symptoms like sleeplessness, memory loss, and vaginal dryness can be helped with estrogen and progesterone therapy.

Your new low progesterone and estrogen levels may also contribute to a shift in insulin sensitivity known as prediabetes or insulin resistance.

reduced progesterone, high and wildly fluctuating estrogen, reduced estrogen, and possibly insulin resistance are the occurrences of perimenopause.

The complete natural perimenopause transition, including four phases plus menopause, takes roughly seven years on average.

very early perimenopause, when cycles are still regular early menopause transition, from the onset of irregular periods late menopause transition, from the first cycle of more than sixty days late perimenopause, which is the twelve months from the final period menopause, which is the life phase that begins one year after your last period.

If you had a partial hysterectomy (uterus removal) but kept your ovaries, you will still go through the four stages of natural perimenopause and have years of 'hidden cycling,' which means years of high estrogen and 'premenstrual' symptoms like mood changes, breast pain, and even endometriosis pain - just no bleed to signal what's going on. It can be a confusing time since you or your doctor may incorrectly believe you are in menopause and attempt to address symptoms of elevated estrogen.

How terrible will things get?

You're probably thinking how awful the perimenopausal symptoms will be at this stage. You may be concerned if you've heard terrifying tales from pals, but your real experience will rely on a variety of things.

If you approach menopause before the age of 45, or if you have surgical or medical menopause, you are more likely to experience symptoms and long-term health problems.

You have a 25% risk of experiencing severe symptoms if you go through a natural perimenopause transition. More than likely, you will experience just minor symptoms, if any at all. If you have no symptoms, rejoice, but keep in mind that you are still in a critical period and should therefore take extra precautions with your health for a few years. If you do experience severe symptoms, it is due to a mix of genetics, your overall health, and the state of your periods prior to perimenopause. Let's take a look at each one separately.

Genetics

The timing of menopause, as well as the types and severity of symptoms, are determined by genetics. If possible, inquire with your mother and older sisters about any family history of heavy periods, night sweats, or sleep issues. Their perimenopausal experience may provide some insight into what you can expect.

Fortunately, genes are only one component of the puzzle. Equally crucial is the expression of those genes, which can be influenced by diet, exercise, and maintaining a healthy circadian rhythm.

Your overall health status

Perimenopause is similar to a health barometer in that it can disclose and exacerbate underlying health conditions. For example, if you are already anxious and not sleeping well, the perimenopausal brain recalibration may make sleep nearly difficult. If you are lacking in the minerals iodine and zinc, the fluctuations in estrogen may present as breast soreness and vaginal dryness, respectively. Finally, if you already have mild insulin resistance, the switch to lower estrogen may cause full insulin resistance and belly weight gain.

'Perimenopause as a health barometer' means that the best treatment for perimenopausal symptoms is frequently the one you needed anyway.

how your periods were before perimenopause

You can generally anticipate an easy perimenopause if you had easy periods because they were a sign that everything was functioning normally, including your body's capacity to eliminate or metabolize estrogen and your brain's capacity to adjust to the natural fluctuations in hormone levels. The same problems that affected your periods will affect your perimenopause, so if you had trouble with your periods, you might also have trouble with it. Unbalanced estrogen metabolism is one instance, which can lead to heavy periods throughout your reproductive years and significantly

heavier periods during perimenopause. Another illustration is neurosteroid change sensitivity, which refers to how sensitively your brain reacts to changes in hormone levels. It can cause both premenstrual and perimenopausal mood symptoms.
Finally, if you continue to use the pill or a combination of oral contraceptives, stopping use may result in "estrogen withdrawal" symptoms.

What follows and maintaining health over the long term

Your primary concern is maintaining good health during what can be a challenging shift. Depending on your circumstance, feeling well may necessitate modifying your food, way of living, and/or taking supplements or hormone therapy, many of which may be short-term solutions. Your health should stabilise as you progress through the menopause, and you may find that you no longer require supplements or hormone therapy to treat your night sweats, mood swings, or sleep issues. Instead, you might need to focus on less severe, persistent symptoms like bladder issues and vaginal dryness.

Chapter 2

Embarrassment, Liberation, Sadness, and all in between

How do you emotionally feel about going through menopause? Or, if you've gone further, about your experience thus far? If you're anything like me, the menopause you eventually go through may not be what you anticipated. Additionally, it's okay if your experience differs from other women's descriptions.

This chapter's main message, if it has one, is that there is no one right way to go through the emotional transition to menopause. You are free to feel happy, sad, or a combination of the two, and that's okay. You are free to express your emotions without having to apologize or justify them. In fact, as we'll see, one of the finest things about second puberty may be the freedom from having to apologize or try to impress others.

Let's start by talking about the stigma of menopause and the embarrassment it may sometimes make us feel, which is what I regard as the "elephant in the room."

Response to aging

First of all, 50 is not old. This is not to argue that growing older is bad because, of course, it's a normal stage of life; however, that is a topic for another book. Since this book is about the menopause and perimenopause, you are probably between the ages of 40 and 60 and could be decades away from retirement. The 'walking stick' style stock photos that are constantly and repeatedly used by the media for articles about menopause serve to reinforce the false association between menopause and old age. It makes sense why my nephew believed that menopause was simply "vaguely about ageing."

Also, ageing is permitted. While not ancient, fifty is not particularly youthful either. Why should we have to? The majority of us are unlikely to look 30 at age 50. We support the ubiquitous and repressive idea that ageing is bad every time we compliment a woman for appearing young, or at least for not looking old. and the need for women to work to maintain their youth and virginity. Which, obviously, we are unable to achieve and ought not to have to do. Instead, we try to stay healthy if we can, strong if we can, and sexually active if that's what we want to do for fun. None of that calls for a certain gaze.

I had personally dreaded losing my youthful beauty and had even frightened it. I believe we might be pardoned for such vanity if you shared my sentiments. Our society constantly promotes the idea that having smooth skin and a slim physique is the only way to be a lady. It was only reasonable for me to fear losing my youthful appearance for this reason, but then something happened. When I turned 50, I realized that I simply care less about appearing young than I had anticipated. I mean, I care about staying healthy, which typically makes me appear a little younger. Yes, I color my hair, but I also care about looking good and dressing nicely. I actually appreciate women who let their natural gray hair alone. Simply put, I simply don't care to fight ageing head-on because, at the end of the day, I have better things to do. It's a welcome change from the continual pressure to look well that many of us experience as young ladies.

As part of a longer-term attempt to let go of perfectionism, it has been a huge relief for me to let go of being the young sort of gorgeous. The idea of perfectionism holds that we may lessen or even completely avoid the hurt of blame, criticism, and shame if we live a perfect life and appear and behave perfectly. A shield, indeed. We carry a twenty-ton shield around with the intention of being protected, but in reality, it is what keeps us from taking flight.

Freedom and obscurity

Patients had told me that menopause was freeing, but I guess I never really believed it. First, if you're heterosexual and worried about that type of thing in the first place, menopausal invisibility is clearly just an issue if you're concerned about being less visible to males, especially younger guys. If you don't color your hair, menopausal invisibility can also make it more difficult to be heard or taken seriously at work. Even though this is terribly unfair, it is true if you work with guys or are in the media. Friends have told me that it's easier to be grey in professions with higher female representation, which makes sense. However, with the recent 'embrace the grey' social media movement, this may all change.

Menopausal invisibility has several positive traits. You are less likely to attract unwanted attention from errant males on the street, which is definitely an improvement, on the men front. If you're anything like me, you might also find that you have more mental space for other things because you're not as worried with potential love interests. It's a sense of liberation from having sexual ideas all the time, like you would have when you were younger. However, this does not preclude you from having sex if you so choose, whether with a partner or by yourself.

since, in fact. It's okay if your libido or sex urge declines. It may be a completely natural reaction to exhaustion from perimenopausal sleep disorder, dropping estrogen levels, or just sexual boredom after 20 or 30 years of marriage, rather than implying that you have a medical condition.

You will no longer be asked if you have children, which is another benefit of menopausal invisibility. If you're like me and didn't have biological children, it's a nice change. Even if you do have children, it would be nice to get a chance to be seen for who you are instead of always being categorized as a mother or not. Freedom from being stared at by strange guys, being preoccupied with sex, and having your reproductive status questioned. On the 'freedom side' of the invisibility-freedom coin, those are but a few perks. The enormous freedom from caring as much as you did about pleasing people is another benefit. Estrogen and progesterone, which are thought to have the impact of making women nicer, gentler, and more selfless, may be at least partially to blame for the need to please that we experience during our reproductive years.

Grief

Grief is a change, sometimes an unwanted change. Grief is the acknowledgment of that shift as well as the loss of a relationship. Grief is love at its core; it is love for what we once had but now no longer have.

Menopause is a phase of life transition, a small amount of grief, and ultimately, a love for the past youth. It's crucial to at least acknowledge the loss we could naturally feel towards the end of our reproductive years, despite how much we might want to "get on with it" and not dwell on bad ideas. I sense it. I'm sorry to have reached the end of my reproductive years and the chance to have biological children, for one thing. Even though I sometimes feel young, I know that I'm not, therefore it's a relief to know that my youth is coming to an end. Even more so when you hear it from other people. In conclusion, it's acceptable to be depressed. unhappy that you're getting older, unhappy that society favors younger ladies more than you, sad that it could be "too late" to do what you intended to do. Of course, many things still have time, but there are certain things for which it is too late; chances have passed you by, just as they have for all of us.

It's also OK to experience sadness for children who have grown up, died, or were never born. As it's acceptable to have sadness over all the other relationships that are altering or ending as you go through life.

Menopause is similar to the start of the autumn, a lovely and fruitful season, but it also marks the beginning of the second half of life, which is when you begin to realize, possibly for the first time, that life is precious and finite. It's not about you in life. Menopause is not either. Instead, menopause and life are a part of the broader and ongoing experiences of countless generations of women.

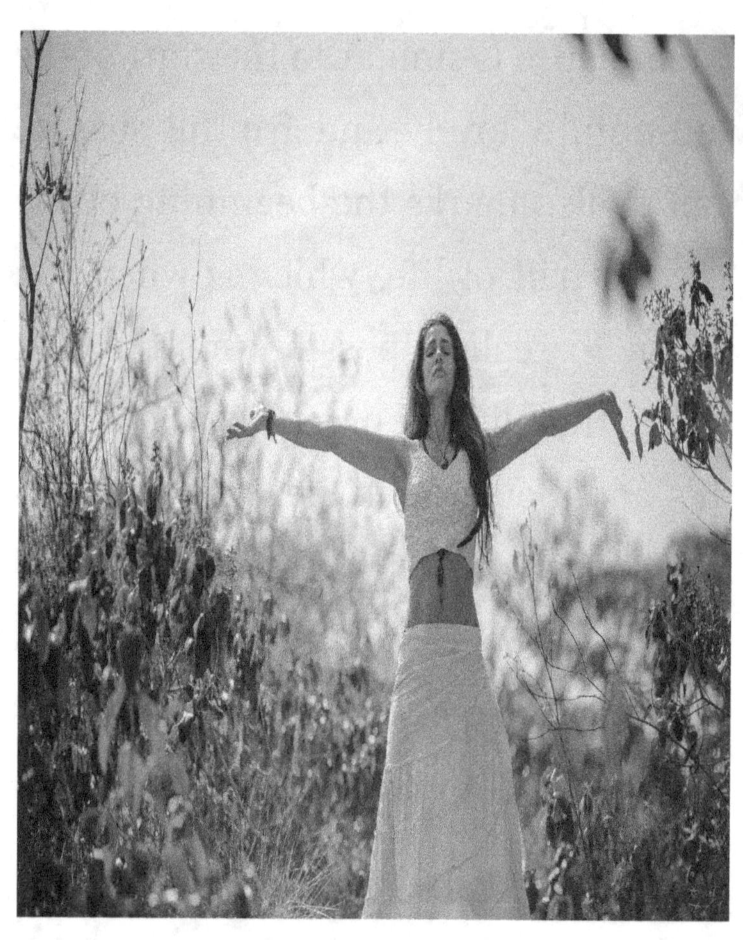

Chapter 3

The Importance Of Natural, Ovulatory Menstrual Cycles

Menopause marks the end of menstrual cycles. However, until you reach menopause, you should try to keep cycling for as long as you can. Why? Because natural menstruation cycles are beneficial. Does that surprise you? You may have been led to believe that menstrual cycles are only for making babies and that once you're done with that, you can take or leave periods. In actuality, menstruation cycles are used to produce hormones as well as infants. With each normal menstrual cycle, you produce a high amount of estrogen (estradiol) in the days preceding ovulation and an even greater amount of progesterone in the two weeks after ovulation. The luteal phase is the two weeks following ovulation, and it is the most important event in the menstrual cycle.

LUTEAL PHASE

The luteal phase is the ideally two-week-long interval between ovulation and the first day of menstrual flow. It is called after the corpus luteum, a transient ovarian gland that produces progesterone and is the only phase during the cycle when large levels of progesterone are produced.

THE OVULATORY CYCLE

An ovulatory cycle is a menstrual cycle that includes ovulation and the production of progesterone.

ANOVULATORY CYCLE

An anovulatory cycle is a menstrual cycle in which no ovulation occurs and so no progesterone is produced.

An anovulatory cycle produces estrogen but does not result in ovulation, hence producing no progesterone. With a too-short luteal phase, you achieve ovulation but do not produce enough progesterone because your luteal phase is too short.

During perimenopause, anovulatory cycles and brief luteal phases are prevalent and can result in complications such as severe bleeding, persistent bleeding, endometrial thickness, and uterine polyps. Other terms for anovulatory cycles include anovulatory bleeding, dysfunctional uterine bleeding, and estrogen dominance.

The crucial thing to remember at this point is that a healthy menstrual cycle is, by definition, an ovulatory cycle that includes estrogen, followed by estrogen plus progesterone. The two hormones collaborate, and their combined effects are numerous.

Estrogen

Estradiol is the estrogen produced during the ovulatory process. It's not your sole estrogen; you also produce estrone in your stomach from adipose (fat) tissue and a variety of estrogen metabolites. Estradiol, on the other hand, is your strongest and best estrogen, and it works with progesterone to achieve many vital things, such as developing muscle and bone and preserving brain and heart health.

Estradiol is also necessary for maintaining a healthy metabolic rate and the ability to shed belly fat. Its metabolic effects arise mostly from how it (in conjunction with progesterone) improves insulin sensitivity and aids in the prevention of insulin resistance and diabetes. After correcting for muscle mass, reproductive-age women have better insulin sensitivity than males, making them less likely to develop insulin resistance and diabetes. This is because estrogen plays a role in this. The 'estrogen advantage' is lost as a woman enters menopause, which raises her risk of insulin resistance and belly fat growth.

Estradiol also makes you want to walk around and exercise more, and it has the potential to reduce your hunger naturally. Because of this, you have less hunger in the days preceding ovulation (when estrogen levels are high) and greater hunger in the final few days before your period (when estradiol levels start to decline). The possible drawback of estrogen is that it might stimulate breast tissue and thicken the uterine lining, which can result in heavy periods, particularly in the early years of perimenopause when you produce more estrogen than usual. You won't experience these undesirable stimulatory effects of estrogen unless you produce enough progesterone to balance it out.

progesterone

The hormone you produce after ovulation is called progesterone, and surprisingly, you produce significantly more progesterone than estrogen. The uterine lining is thinned by progesterone, which counteracts estrogen's thickening of the uterine lining and can lessen the frequency of heavy periods. Progesterone also has the advantage of calming the brain, which can help with anxiety reduction and sleep promotion. Additionally, progesterone lowers inflammation, normalizes immunological function, strengthens bones, safeguards the heart, boosts metabolism, and may lower the risk of breast cancer.

You will eventually cease ovulating and lose practically all of your progesterone as a result of perimenopause. Contrast that with estrogen, which is still produced by the enzyme aromatase during menopause and is only somewhat reduced during perimenopause.

Ovulation improves wellbeing

Even years after you approach menopause and produce less estrogen and no progesterone, your lifelong cumulative exposure to both estrogen and progesterone is advantageous. Osteoporosis, breast cancer, and heart disease can all be prevented throughout the perimenopausal years with regular menstrual cycles and consistently normal ovulation, and she mostly credits progesterone for this effect. Progesterone gradually strengthens bones, safeguards the breasts, and contributes to the development of a healthier, more resilient physiology cycle by cycle. Therefore, every ovulatory cycle acts as a deposit into the health-related bank account. The same cannot be stated for every cycle of hormonal birth control using progestins.

Chapter 4

Second puberty's hormonal and physiological changes

In this chapter, we'll look at the physiological changes that occur throughout perimenopause and menopause as well as the wide range of symptoms that may appear. You will transition from high, fluctuating estrogen combined with low or no progesterone during the initial stages of natural perimenopause to low estrogen and no progesterone by the time you reach menopause. In addition to menopause, these changes take place over four phases: very early perimenopause, when cycles are still regular early menopause transition, from the start of irregular periods of late menopause transition, from the first cycle lasting more than sixty days late perimenopause, which lasts for twelve months after the last period, and menopause, which is the stage of life that starts one year after your last period.

Progesterone decline

Making estrogen is much simpler than making progesterone. This is because estrogen is produced during the process of ovulation, and as we saw with anovulatory cycles, it is possible to produce significant amounts of estrogen without ever reaching ovulation.

Progesterone, on the other hand, is only produced after ovulation, which is unfortunately challenging. Even when you were young and had active ovarian follicles, ovulation was challenging. The ability to ovulate back then required several different elements, including normal thyroid function and optimal insulin sensitivity. Now, in perimenopause, you still require all of those things (good thyroid, insulin, and so on), but you now have to contend with the extra difficulty that your follicles are simply less active or responsive. That is why you are currently experiencing anovulatory periods and producing little or no progesterone.

The problem is caused by a lack of progesterone. Many perimenopausal symptoms, such as headaches, breast pain, and heavy periods, are caused by the loss of progesterone while still having a lot of estrogen (perhaps even more estrogen).

Anovulatory cycles
hormone imbalance
estrogen and progesterone imbalance
dysfunctional uterine hemorrhage
ovulatory dysfunction
unopposed estrogen
estrogen dominance
are all terms for the combination of high estrogen and low or no progesterone.

The last time you had high estrogen and no progesterone was when you were in first puberty when your hormonal system was still evolving. Because you had anovulatory cycles back then, you may have experienced symptoms of unopposed estrogen, such as migraines and heavy periods. When you lose progesterone, you will notice that the hormone influences several parts of health, including the immune system and, most critically, the brain. When you lose progesterone, you have to re-calibrate those systems (particularly the brain), and if that goes well, you should be fine. If things don't go as planned, you may experience one or more of the following symptoms.

Mood and sleep disruption

Progesterone deficiency alters the brain and nerve system, reducing your ability to cope with stress. It also increases the risk of anxiety, depression, memory loss, and sleep disturbance, all of which can lead to chronic physical discomfort if left untreated. Histamine or mast cell activation can similarly alter the mood symptoms of early perimenopause.

Night sweats and hot flushes

When you're still producing a lot of estrogen but no progesterone, hot flushes and night sweats can start early in perimenopause. Unfortunately, if flushes begin early (while you are still having regular periods), they can last for up to ten years. If flushes start later (after the final period), they will probably persist for only a year or two.

Heart palpitations

The term "heart palpitations" refers to the sense of a skipped heartbeat as well as a pounding or fluttering heartbeat. It is a frequent and unpleasant perimenopausal symptom that can be accompanied by hot flushes, temporarily raising heart rate by as much as sixteen beats per minute.

Migraines

Perimenopause is connected with high and fluctuating levels of both estrogen and histamine, two significant contributors to migraines, which can cause an increase in migraine frequency because the brain is deprived of progesterone's beneficial calming impact.

Immune disorder

When the immune system attacks the body's tissues, it is referred to as an autoimmune illness or autoimmunity. Because of the significant immune system remodeling brought on by the loss of progesterone and estrogen, some autoimmune diseases are more prevalent during perimenopause and early menopause. Hashimoto's thyroid disease is the most prevalent autoimmune condition.

Period pain and heavy periods

Progesterone reduces menstrual flow, thins the uterine lining, and lessens period pain. Because of this, you're more likely to have painful and heavy periods throughout the first and second puberty (when progesterone levels are low).

High and erratic estrogen levels

Contrary to what you may have heard, estrogen levels during perimenopause do not likely fall gradually. It might be, in which case your periods will gradually get lighter. It's more likely that your estrogen levels will increase by up to three times from when you were younger. Heavy periods, breast soreness, and irritability can be signs of high, variable estrogen, whereas sadness and night sweats can be signs of low estrogen.

Angry mood

High, erratic estrogen levels can also contribute to irritability, intense wrath, and sleeplessness. The way estrogen stimulates mast cells and histamine can lead to several issues, including anxiety, heavy periods, migraines, hives, hay fever, and other symptoms.

Losing estrogen

We've looked at the high, variable estrogen of the earlier periods of perimenopause, which can also create symptoms from falling estrogen or withdrawal from high to low. Let's now enter the realm of consistently decreased estrogen, which starts the day after your last period. 'Lower estrogen' does not mean 'no estrogen,' as you will always have some estrogen, but not as much as before. During menopause, your ovaries will still produce some estradiol (about 10% of what you used to make), and an enzyme called aromatase will produce it throughout the rest of your body. Aromatase transforms the androgens testosterone and androstenedione into the estrogens estradiol and estrone and does so in every unique cell of every tissue. Local estrogen production enables organs like the heart and brain to produce only the amount of estrogen they require. As a result, they receive some estrogen (which is necessary) while also being protected against the negative consequences of too much. Intracrinology, or carefully controlled local estrogen production, is crucial for men, women, and children.

Local cell intracrinology is the main source of estrogen for both men and children. The enormous amount of estradiol produced by the ovaries is more important for women of reproductive age than the estrogen from intracrinology. After menopause, intracrinology resumes control when ovarian estrogen production declines.

Your body 'dials up' estrogen during menopause by 1) boosting aromatase activity and 2) increasing the production of androgens such androstenedione from the ovaries and DHEA (dehydroepiandrosterone) from the adrenal glands. You can promote the intracrinological process and preserve a healthy level of intracellular estrogen by keeping a healthy level of DHEA.

By changing the quantity and sensitivity of estrogen receptors, which serve as estrogen's docking stations, your body can increase estrogen in three different ways. Your body might magnify the signal of your new decreased estrogen level by making estrogen receptors more sensitive. The duration of menopausal symptoms may be related to how long it takes to upregulate aromatase and activate estrogen receptors.

In general, aromatase upregulation is advantageous because it gives you the constant supply of estrogen that you require. In addition, excessive estrone production in menopausal years is a risk factor for cardiovascular disease, fibroids, pelvic pain, irregular uterine bleeding, and breast cancer. Estrone is produced by the enzyme aromatase in abdominal adipose (fat) tissue. Another reason to recognize and treat insulin resistance is high abdominal adipose aromatase activity, which is typically caused by it. Let's now look at the symptoms related to reduced or falling estrogen.

Night sweats and hot flashes

It is preferable to use progesterone to treat hot flashes and night sweats that start during perimenopause because they are caused by low progesterone and variable estrogen. If flushes persist after the last period, they are more likely the result of less estrogen, albeit it is still changing, and they can be treated with estrogen plus progesterone.

Sleep and mood disruption

As we have already shown, low progesterone, high estrogen, and mast cell activation, or histamine, are the causes of mood symptoms in the early stages of perimenopause. In the early years of menopause and the latter stages of perimenopause mood problems are brought on by a change in the brain's energy system brought on by reduced estrogen.

Vaginal dryness

The tissues of the vagina, vulva, and urethra can thin as a result of low estrogen levels. One of the few menopause symptoms that is permanent rather than passing, it is known as vaginal atrophy or the genitourinary syndrome of menopause

(GSM). Dryness, discomfort, itching, increased frequency of urination, incontinence, prolapse, and increased susceptibility to urinary tract infections (UTIs) are some of the symptoms.

Pains in the body

In some studies, hot flushes are not as common a symptom of menopause as aching muscles and joints. It's not unusual to be diagnosed with fibromyalgia during perimenopause and the first years of menopause, most likely as a result of sleep disturbances and the loss of progesterone and estrogen's natural anti-inflammatory effects.

Weight gain in the abdomen

Finally, reduced estrogen and progesterone levels can produce a metabolic shift that contributes to belly fat growth. A few things are going on. For starters, you're losing estradiol's anabolic characteristics, which means you're losing muscle mass, which lowers metabolism. You're also losing estrogen's and progesterone's anti-inflammatory and metabolism-stimulating effects, which can contribute to insulin resistance, a major theme in this book. Menopause increases your chance of insulin resistance, and insulin resistance might exacerbate menopausal symptoms. Part of the problem stems from the natural transition to relative androgen excess that occurs throughout perimenopause and menopause.

If you previously had the hormonal disease PCOS, menopausal insulin resistance and weight gain are more common. This is because PCOS is characterized by androgen excess and insulin resistance, both of which tend to progress and worsen with menopause (in the absence of treatment).

Perimenopause diagnosis

There is no blood test for perimenopause, and measuring estrogen and progesterone levels is usually not worth the effort. Perimenopause is instead diagnosed based on symptoms and context.

A midlife woman with regular cycles is likely to be in perimenopause if she experiences three of the nine changes listed below:

new heavy beginning and/or longer flow Menstrual cycles of 25 days or less breasts that are aching, puffy, or lumpy for the first time

new waking up in the middle of the night

Menstrual cramps have become quite severe.

Premenstrually new or significantly increased migraine headaches, new or increased premenstrual mood swings, and weight gain without changes in diet or exercise are some of the symptoms of the onset of night sweats. In other words, if you are above 35 and exhibit at least three of these symptoms, you are probably going through perimenopause.

On the other hand, menopause is the life stage that starts a year after your last menstruation. A blood test for FSH can be used to identify early or premature menopause, which we'll talk about later.

When perimenopause occurs
Four phases make up the procedure's average duration of seven years.

1   **Exceptionally   early perimenopause**
During this phase, your menstrual cycle is still regular, however, it may

be shorter (21–26 days). Your progesterone levels are probably lower than they once were, but your estrogen levels are higher, which puts you at risk for migraines, insomnia, heavier periods, and increased period pain. Normally, this phase lasts between two and five years.

2 Transition into the early menopause

Your cycle is beginning to vary in length by more than seven days when calculating from day 1 to day 1. You still have high, fluctuating estrogen and low progesterone, just like in the earlier phase, but now, when your estrogen drops, it becomes even lower, which may lead to worsening hot flashes and night sweats. Two to three years pass between the start of irregular cycles and the first skipped period.

3 Transition into late menopause

You now experience your first missed period or cycle that lasts more than 60 days. Breast discomfort should subside, but hot flushes and night sweats may worsen and you may still get one or two very heavy periods. It should take you four years from this point until you reach menopause, which will occur 12 months following your last period.

4 Postmenopausal women

When you believe that your last period has passed and you still have a year to go before menopause, you are in late perimenopause. You should start to experience fewer symptoms of high, fluctuating estrogen, such as migraines and mood disorders, as this is the start of the adjustment to lower estrogen. Unless you start having periods again, in which case your estrogen levels may rise once again and some of those symptoms may come back. The likelihood of getting another period increases with age, and if you do, you'll have to restart the countdown to menopause. From this point on, hot flushes could last for a year or longer.

Menopause

The life stage that starts a year following your last menstruation is called menopause. In conclusion, perimenopause starts with brief cycles and heavy bleeding, progresses to extended cycles and light bleeding, and finally results in a year without bleeding.

The four phases only relate to menopause, which normally occurs in women in their late forties or early fifties, as was previously stated. They do not apply to menopause brought on by basic ovarian insufficiency or to menopause brought on by medical or surgical procedures.

Early menopause and its effects

'Early menopause' or primary ovarian insufficiency

Primary ovarian insufficiency (POI), also known as premature ovarian failure, premature menopause, or early menopause, is the cause of menopause before the age of 40. It differs from menopause in that it results from ovarian dysfunction. Some specialists claim that POI often happens relatively suddenly, without the series of perimenopausal events mentioned above, and that it can be accompanied by more severe symptoms. Before periods cease, POI can also cause mood swings and severe bleeding.

Primary ovarian insufficiency affects roughly one in 100 women and is identified by two high FSH levels (greater than 40 IU/L) at least a month apart. Genetics, autoimmune disorders, and chemotherapy or radiation therapy are risk factors. The cause is typically unknown.

Pregnancy in people with primary ovarian insufficiency is uncommon but not impossible. According to a thorough assessment of the literature,

5–10% of women with POI go on to become pregnant naturally.

You'll probably need menopausal hormone therapy to manage your symptoms and lower your long-term risk of dementia, heart disease, and osteoporosis.

Surgical Menopause

When your ovaries stop functioning as a result of medical or surgical treatment, this is known as medical or induced menopause. The most frequent causes include chemo, radiation, or surgical ovarian removal during a total hysterectomy. Normal menopause is not caused by medical or surgical procedures. One of the effects is that hormone levels drop more quickly, which might lead to sensations that are exceptionally intense, notably hot flashes. Because you won't have the ongoing supply of estrogen and androgens provided by functional menopausal ovaries, it's also linked to an exceptionally low level of hormones. Hormone therapy can help to reduce but not eliminate the danger of low hormones, which could increase your long-term risk of osteoporosis, heart disease, and dementia. Due to this, the majority of medical professionals now advise against removing ovaries unless there is a very significant risk of ovarian cancer.

Are the signs of menopause a byproduct of contemporary life?

Menopause has existed for as long as humans have, and it's possible that it was the catalyst for the evolution of a longer human lifetime.

Menopausal symptoms, however, are not common in human civilization even if menopause is. For instance, modern forager women report few (or rarely any) negative symptoms and typically see menopause as a good thing. Many of those same women go on to age healthily and contentedly, which somewhat refutes the idea that losing estrogen is the start of diseases.

What is happening? Is it feasible that, save from certain circumstances, losing estrogen is not a significant deal? If so, what exactly is that "something else"? What element or elements of contemporary life predispose us to menopausal symptoms? There are several opposing influences.

The first is the comparatively smaller amount of time we spend carrying a child or nursing a baby. This is especially true in the years leading up to menopause when the majority of us have either not had any pregnancies or have had only a few, but many years earlier. In contrast, women in forager societies will typically have put in many more total years, including the years preceding menopause, while they were expecting or nursing a child. As a result, they skip the high, fluctuating estrogen and subsequent "estrogen withdrawal" of modern perimenopause, and instead experience menopause as a smooth transition from the low estrogen state of breastfeeding to the equally low estrogen state of menopause.

Another more concerning idea is that at least some menopause symptoms and health hazards, including mood issues, may be linked to the poisonous lead released from bones during the normal, accelerated bone loss associated with menopause. In the modern world, lead steadily builds up in the bones over a lifetime, particularly in women who were exposed to greater amounts, including those who lived in a home constructed before 1960. There hasn't been a lot of research, but other environmental contaminants may influence menopause symptoms and perhaps its timing.

All of the contemporary issues, such as the disturbance of circadian rhythm, chronic inflammation, poor microbiota, and, most critically, insulin resistance, could also increase our susceptibility to menopausal symptoms. Menopause raises the likelihood of insulin resistance, as we learned earlier in this chapter, and insulin resistance can also make menopause symptoms worse. Women in ancient foraging societies consume foods low in calories and sugar, which lowers their risk of developing insulin resistance and menopausal symptoms.

Can the menopause be postponed?

The quick response is no, not at this time. Based on heredity, the menopause's timing is predetermined. There is no known technique to delay it, however, illness or smoking can bring it a little earlier.

Of course, if medicine finds a means to keep the ovaries active for additional years or perhaps decades, that could alter. The likelihood that ovaries do not run out of eggs and instead contain ovarian stem cells, which can theoretically be induced to expand and produce new follicles or eggs, makes such a situation plausible.

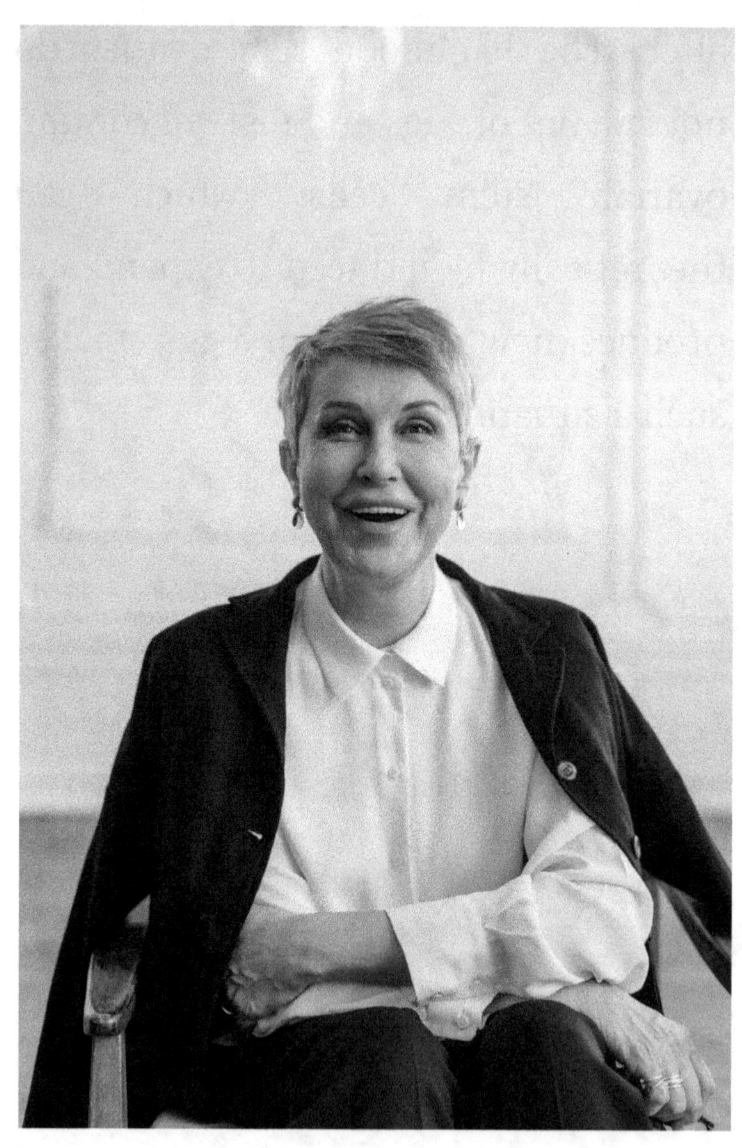

Chapter 5

Perimenopause and beyond: general maintenance

Relax your nervous system

Losing progesterone and subsequently estrogen might be unsettling for your brain and nerve system. They must recalibrate to adapt, and this process necessitates a certain level of overall health and resilience. So the first step in general maintenance is to improve the health and resilience of your nervous system. This will make you feel better now and increase your chances of staying well in the long run. Remember that perimenopause is a vital period for overall health and the neurological system in particular. Managing your stress now may help you avoid mood difficulties later.

To understand your nervous system, you must first understand three components of it: your autonomic nervous system, your hypothalamic-pituitary-adrenal (HPA) axis, and your circadian rhythm. Let's take a look at each one separately.

Autonomic Nervous system

The autonomic nervous system is responsible for unconscious body activities such as breathing, digestion, and heartbeat. Depending on whether part of the autonomic system is engaged, it plays a significant role in both responding to and recovering from stress.

The sympathetic nervous system, which is related to the neurotransmitters adrenaline and noradrenaline and increases respiration, pulse, and alertness, is the half that increases the sense of stress. It is beneficial to have some sympathetic activity or tone because it allows you to respond to unanticipated difficulties or demands. Too much sympathetic tone can lead to persistent hyperarousal or tension, which is bad for your sleep, brain, and hormone system.

The parasympathetic nervous system, which is related to the hormone oxytocin and the neurotransmitter acetylcholine and lowers respiration, pulse, and alertness, is the half of the autonomic nervous system that reduces stress. Parasympathetic activity or tone encourages processes that the body prefers to perform when at rest, such as sleep, healthy digestion, and healing.

Consider measuring your heart rate variability (HRV), which is the extent to which the intervals between heartbeats fluctuate from one heartbeat to the next, if you want an easy approach to check your parasympathetic tone. You can measure it using a Bluetooth heart-rate monitor and an app for your smartphone.

Higher heart rate variability is beneficial since it is related to increased parasympathetic tone. True, your heart is pounding less frequently, which sounds negative, but it implies that your parasympathetic nervous system is in charge and is responding to your breath and other stimuli by adjusting your heart rate. Healthy heart rate variability indicates that your nervous system is in a state of resilience.

The vagus nerve, a cranial nerve that communicates directly from the brain to the body, is a major factor in heart rate variability and parasympathetic tone. Such direct contact is analogous to a high-speed fiber-optic cable connecting your brain and body, allowing your brain to monitor your physical status minutely and determine if everything is in order.

Diet and lifestyle changes to boost parasympathetic tone

You may soothe your vagus nerve and parasympathetic nervous system by sending it calm and safe messages like the ones below:

Get outside and enjoy nature. Walking in nature (green exercise) boosts parasympathetic tone both immediately after the activity and hours later when sleeping.

Make new social relationships.
Regular social connection, whether with a partner, family, friends, or even a pet, boosts the release of oxytocin, engages the vagus nerve, and enhances heart rate variability.

Experiment with extended exhalations as a breathing technique.
Slowing your breath and exhaling slowly activates the vagus nerve, which

soothes the sympathetic fight-or-flight stress response.

Yoga. Slow exhales are an important aspect of yoga, and Stress-Proof: the scientific answer to protect your brain and body, yoga has a few extra advantages. Poses with the hands over the head stimulate blood pressure sensors in the neck and chest, signaling the brain to switch between sympathetic and parasympathetic nervous systems. When combined with the practice of silence, this has a top-down effect.

The autonomic nervous system and the stress response are both regulated. Traditional hatha yoga's slow pace has been demonstrated to improve heart rate variability and parasympathetic tone.

This is just one of several strategies for improving the health of the autonomic nervous system. Bitter foods, massage or bodywork, exposure to cold water, and maintaining good gut microbes are among the others.

HPA (hypothalamic-pituitary-adrenal) axis

The HPA axis, which communicates between the brain (hypothalamus and pituitary gland) and the adrenal glands or stress glands, is closely related to the autonomic nervous system. If you've ever heard the terms 'adrenal tiredness' or 'adrenal exhaustion,' you'll understand what I mean.

The right medical word for the entire system that includes the adrenal glands is the HPA axis, and the correct phrase for a reduced ability to cope with stress is HPA axis dysfunction or dysregulation.

When your HPA axis is working properly, you create higher levels of the stress hormones cortisol and adrenaline only when needed and then turn them off again.

When your HPA axis is dysfunctional, you produce chronically elevated levels of cortisol and adrenaline, which can contribute to depression, insomnia, fatigue, decreased muscle mass, low libido, impaired immune function, and insulin resistance. All of these symptoms are related to menopause.

The other link between HPA axis failure and menopause is that it is related to lower levels of the adrenal hormone DHEA, which, as you may recall from the previous chapter, is the precursor to intracrine or local estrogen production with aromatase. As a result, taking action to optimize the functioning of your HPA axis can aid in the production of estrogen during menopause.

Chronic stress, as well as undereating, illness, vitamin deficiencies, sleep deprivation, and disruption of the circadian rhythm, can all lead to HPA axis dysfunction. Perimenopause can potentially produce HPA axis dysfunction because progesterone generally helps to improve HPA axis function.

As you approach perimenopause, you may become more prone to HPA axis dysfunction as a result of persistent stress and other causes. In consequence, HPA axis dysfunction can exacerbate or cause numerous perimenopausal and menopausal symptoms.

HPA axis dysfunction testing

There is no good means to test for HPA axis dysfunction at this time. A recent study examined all available approaches, including salivary cortisol, and determined that none of them are reliable predictors of exhaustion or symptoms. Better testing methods may become available in the future, but in the meantime, I assess HPA axis impairment based on sleeplessness and morning fatigue symptoms.

Diet and lifestyle changes can help to control the HPA axis.

Using the parasympathetic nervous system to stabilize and control the HPA axis is a great technique to do so. That includes all of the measures we just described, such as getting outside, practicing breathing techniques, and doing yoga.

Doing more of what you enjoy and promoting a healthy circadian rhythm are two other options. Maintaining a healthy HPA axis may also necessitate more rest, which I understand is difficult in our fast-paced society. A hectic schedule can trap you in a state of busyness that is simply unsuitable for a healthy HPA axis. Your body requires you to slow down, and if you can't find a method to do so, your body will. Maintaining steady blood sugar is one of the finest nutritional approaches to aid your HPA axis. This includes eliminating desserts and consuming protein at every meal, especially breakfast.

Several nutritional supplements, including B vitamins and magnesium, can help to regulate the HPA axis.

The Circadian rhythm

Every cell in your body has a 'clock' and operates on a 24-hour cycle. Maintaining that routine is a fantastic approach to optimize overall health, including metabolism, emotions, sleep, bones, and, of course, the HPA axis.

The suprachiasmatic nucleus of the brain serves as the master clock for all of your body clocks, acting as the lead metronome, keeping all of your clocks in sync. It accomplishes this by synchronizing the release of numerous neuronal and hormonal signals, such as cortisol from the HPA axis and melatonin from the pineal gland. Cortisol is your daytime or daylight hormone, whereas melatonin is your nighttime or darkness hormone. Melatonin promotes sleep as well as supporting healthy digestion, immunological function, and metabolism.

Doing things at the wrong time, like eating or being exposed to blue light throughout the night, is the quickest way to upset your circadian rhythm. If you've ever looked after a child or a pet, you know how much they want to have a routine. Your body is the same, so please provide it with what it requires when it requires it. Because the suprachiasmatic nucleus is sensitive to both progesterone and estrogen, perimenopause can impair circadian rhythm. Another system has to be re-calibrated.

A healthy circadian rhythm can be achieved by diet and lifestyle changes.

Light in the morning and darkness at night. Blue-wavelength light is most intense in the morning and least intense in the evening. Blue light signals your brain it's daytime, which is useful when it's daytime, especially in the morning. Try starting your day outside, perhaps with an early walk, which provides both morning light and healthful green activity. Dimming your screen, donning blue-blocking glasses, or limiting screen time an hour or two before bedtime are all simple options.

Protein in the morning. Eating protein before 10 a.m. provides positive signals to the 'clock genes' that control insulin and metabolism. As a result, breakfast protein can aid in regulating circadian rhythm and support weight loss. Even if you're following an intermittent fasting regimen (described later), attempt to have at least a small dish of protein by 10 a.m. Reduce your intake of alcohol. Melatonin levels are reduced by alcohol, which can disturb the circadian cycle. That is one of the reasons to consider lowering or eliminating alcohol consumption. We'll go over alcohol in further detail later in the chapter.

Bathe in warm water. A warm bath or shower an hour or two before going to bed will help you fall and remain asleep. It works by momentarily boosting your body temperature and then allowing it to drop again, making you sleepy. A bath in the afternoon, on the other hand, can help to normalize the circadian rhythm and enhance mood.

Melatonin. Melatonin is a sleep aid that works in part by reducing core body temperature and promoting circadian rhythm.

To summarize, keeping the nervous system healthy necessitates methods for the autonomic nervous system, the HPA axis, and the circadian rhythm. Fortunately, many of the same common-sense solutions apply to all three. Following that, we'll go through all of the methods you may use to lessen chronic inflammation.

Reduce inflammation

Chronic inflammation must be reduced as part of a healthy perimenopause transition because untreated chronic inflammation makes everything more difficult. Chronic inflammation, for example, can trigger the sympathetic nervous system, which causes hot flushes. Chronic inflammation is also harmful to mood and sleep, and it can make periods heavier. Finally, persistent inflammation might aggravate insulin resistance and menopausal weight gain.

What precisely is chronic inflammation? In basic terms, it is the chronic, long-term activation of the immune system. It is distinct from acute inflammation, which is the short-term activation of the immune system to heal a wound or protect against infection.

Chemical messengers produced by your immune system are involved in chronic inflammation. You don't need to know the names of these proteins, which include TNF-alpha, IL-6, and IL-8. I'll just call them inflammatory cytokines or inflammation.

What is the source of chronic inflammation?

Anything that excites, stresses, or hinders immune function might cause chronic inflammation. It could be as easy as junk food, a lack of sleep, or chronic emotional stress. It could also be more complicated concerns, such as Epstein-Barr virus infection or autoimmune disease.

Inflammation can also be caused by something as simple as smoking. Cigarette smoke contains cadmium, pesticides, and other hormone-damaging, immune-activating chemicals, making it one of the most inflammatory things you can do, as well as one of the few lifestyle factors that has been proven to accelerate menopause. If you smoke, your first step should be to discover a means to stop.

Finally, persistent inflammation can be caused by insulin resistance, digestive issues, or exposure to environmental pollutants. Let's take a look at each one separately.

Insulin sensitivity

Simply put, insulin resistance is characterized by chronically high levels of insulin, the hormone that stimulates cells to absorb glucose. It's also known as hyperinsulinemia, metabolic syndrome, or prediabetes, and it affects one out of every two people. If left untreated, insulin resistance might progress to type 2 diabetes. The issue with insulin resistance is not insulin itself, which is, of course, a necessary and beneficial hormone. Insulin benefits include converting food into energy (necessary for living), encouraging muscle growth (anabolic), and aiding in the maintenance of a healthy menstrual cycle. Undereating might lead young women to miss their periods due to low insulin levels.

The problem with insulin resistance is underlying metabolic dysfunction, which results in a diminished ability of the cells to respond to insulin, resulting in a compensatory rise in insulin. High insulin is thus a symptom of underlying metabolic dysfunction as well as a source of reduced metabolic flexibility, which implies that cells have a reduced ability to switch from utilizing glucose for energy to using ketones, which are a metabolite of glucose.

High insulin levels are also a cause of inflammation, leading to a type of inflammation known as meta-inflammation, which is short for "metabolic inflammation." Untreated, insulin resistance, metabolic inflexibility, and meta-inflammation can lead to a variety of poor long-term health effects, including abdominal weight increase and the following:

Memory loss symptoms of excessive androgens, such as facial hair, and various types of hair loss High cholesterol raises the long-term risk of osteoporosis, heart disease, and dementia.

uterine fibroids cause hot flushes Anovulatory hemorrhage and thicker uterine lining.

Insulin resistance contributes to uterine lining thickening in part through upregulating the enzyme aromatase, which we encountered in the previous chapter. This results in higher levels of estrone, which can contribute to irregular uterine bleeding, adenomyosis, fibroids, and an increased risk of breast cancer.

Symptoms of insulin resistance and risk factors

Do you suffer from insulin resistance? Are you certain?

The most common symptom of insulin resistance is abdominal weight gain, often known as apple-shaped weight increase or weight gain around the midsection or upper torso.

It is also possible to have insulin resistance without experiencing any noticeable abdominal weight gain, which is why it is critical to test for and examine other signs and symptoms such as fatigue, sugar cravings, high triglycerides, high cholesterol, skin tags, and acanthosis nigricans, a dark, velvety discoloration of the skin in the armpits, groin, and neck folds.

A familial history of diabetes or a personal history of gestational diabetes or PCOS are also risk factors for insulin resistance.

Insulin resistance testing

The insulin resistance test is a test for the hormone insulin, not for glucose. In other words, normal blood sugar or glucose levels cannot rule out insulin resistance. Insulin testing can be done as a 'fasting insulin' test or an 'oral glucose tolerance test (GTT) with insulin,' which involves taking a fasting blood sample and then drinking a glucose drink before taking two further samples at one- and two-hour intervals. If you're going to have a glucose tolerance test, it's far better to have it 'with insulin' so you can see your insulin levels as well. Insulin resistance is an important consideration in perimenopause and menopause because 1) underlying insulin resistance can worsen practically any symptom and 2) the natural testosterone dominance of menopause might worsen insulin resistance. Insulin resistance, fortunately, can be corrected with measures such as intermittent fasting, activity, and enough protein consumption.

Digestive wellness

Fixing digestive issues is a crucial element of lowering chronic inflammation because they are another source of inflammation. Please keep in mind that your immune system and digestion are, in some ways, one continuous entity when it comes to 'digestive' inflammation. For example, 80% of your immune system is centered on digestion, where it is constantly in contact with your stomach and gut flora.

As a result, anything wrong with your stomach or gut flora might trigger your immune system and create inflammation.

Food sensitivities, intestinal permeability, and issues with the gut bacteria or microbiome are all things that might go wrong with digestion.

Food intolerances

A food sensitivity or intolerance develops when food upsets your gut bacteria or inflames your gut lining, causing your immune system to become activated. Food sensitivity encompasses any negative reaction to a food and is a larger, more nuanced reaction than food allergy. Headaches, joint discomfort, intestinal bloating, and food cravings are all symptoms of sensitivity, and many of these can be linked to other causes, making it a fairly contentious topic. Any item can potentially cause a food sensitivity reaction, however, wheat and dairy products are the most typically reactive foods.

Diet and lifestyle changes to promote gut health

Reduce your consumption of alcohol because it can harm your microbiome.

Consume vegetables and nutritious carbohydrates since they nourish beneficial bacteria. Avoid ultra-processed foods since they deplete beneficial microbes.

Concentrated sugar should be avoided because it can nourish unfavorable microbes.

Identify food sensitivities, such as wheat and dairy, and avoid them if they are causing inflammation.

Determine whether you have a sensitivity to high-amine or nickel-containing foods and eliminate them if they are causing inflammation.

Stress should be managed because it causes dysbiosis.

Exercise benefits the health of the gut microbiome.

Get adequate sleep because it helps to maintain a healthy microbiota.

Maintain appropriate stomach acid since it aids in the reduction of unfavorable bacteria. If you have digestive bloating and heartburn, it could be due to low (rather than high) stomach acid, which could be improved with betaine HCl.

Avoid drugs that harm gut microorganisms as much as possible. This includes birth control pills, antibiotics, and stomach acid medicines.

Environmental Toxins

Toxins in the environment, such as solvents, plastics, pesticides, or toxic metals like lead, can cause inflammation. I saved this issue for last because 1) avoiding toxins may not be as crucial as other aspects like eating veggies to support your microbiota, and 2) avoiding toxins can be difficult.

Toxins, on the other hand, are worth considering because they can cause problems such as: accelerating menopause, stimulating fibroid growth, contributing to perimenopausal symptoms, and increasing the risk of long-term problems such as thyroid disease, insulin resistance, weight gain, and heart disease.

Reduce your exposure.

We are all exposed to toxins, so until our governments pass stricter regulations or the existing regulations take effect, we must make the best of a terrible situation and strive to limit our exposure. You cannot avoid all toxins and can only make rational, evident choices when they are available. For example, if you can afford it, buy organic food; if you can't, don't worry; eating non-organic vegetables is preferable to eating no vegetables at all.

Avoid chemicals used in agricultural, gardening, and building materials as much as possible, and limit your exposure to needless household items such as air fresheners, dryer sheets, waterproofing chemicals, stain repellents, and carpet cleaners. Use an activated-carbon water filter to eliminate chlorine from your drinking water, avoid phthalate-containing cosmetics, and always wash your hands after handling thermal paper cash-register receipts, which are high in BPA.

You can also take the simple step of attempting to keep harmful residues from entering your home. This includes removing your outside shoes, cleaning up dust regularly, and getting rid of carpets, which collect dust and residue.

Diet and lifestyle changes to promote healthy toxin elimination

Detoxification is the most important and energy-intensive action that your cells perform every minute of every day. To put it another way, your body is designed to detoxify.

To aid your body's natural detoxification process, try the following:

Maintaining a healthy gut microbiota is important because it aids in the elimination of toxins through your stools.

Food sensitivities should be identified and avoided since they can promote inflammation in the gut, which inhibits helpful detoxification.

Get plenty of rest because deep sleep is when your detoxifying mechanisms are at their most active.

Sweat in the sauna or while exercising to mobilize and remove toxins. Make sure to stay hydrated.

Consider taking sulforaphane, N-acetyl cysteine, selenium, or glycine, which can help to upregulate good detoxification pathways. Selenium and glycine are very beneficial for the proper elimination of harmful lead. Reduce or reduce your consumption of alcohol because it hinders your body's ability to detoxify.

Feed your body

A good diet is essential for navigating the perimenopause transition. In this section, we'll look at all of the nutrients you need to keep healthy, beginning with protein.

Protein

Protein contains the amino acids required for, well, everything. Every cell in the body, including the digestive system, immune system, and brain, requires amino acids for repair and maintenance. Amino acids also aid in maintaining strong muscles and bones, which is especially important during menopause, when decreasing estrogen levels can cause muscle and bone density loss.

To maintain muscle mass as a menopausal woman, you'll need a little more protein than you did when you were younger. In practice, what does that look like? You probably needed at least 1 gram of protein per kilogram of ideal body weight per day when you were younger. For example, if your ideal weight is 65 kilograms, you used to require roughly 65 grams of protein per day, which translates to 22 grams of high-quality protein with each meal. Menopause necessitates closer to 1.2 grams per kilogram per day, or 78 grams altogether, which is 26 grams per meal or 20 grams per meal with a protein snack or supplement. If you engage in high-intensity exercise or have insulin resistance, you will require even more protein to repair muscle and replace protein lost due to insulin resistance.

There are a few things to keep in mind if you only eat plant protein.

To get 20 grams of protein, for example, you'll need 242 grams of chickpeas versus 87 grams of chicken. Second, combining grains and pulses will provide you with a comprehensive array of all nine essential amino acids. You may also need to supplement the amino acids leucine and taurine, which are difficult to obtain from plant protein.

Carbohydrates and fat

The energy macronutrients you can change depending on your exercise level and if you're trying to lose weight are fat and carbohydrates. For example, if you're more active, you'll require more energy, and hence more fat and carbohydrates; if you're less active or trying to lose weight, you'll require less.

Of course, you want some fat and carbohydrates because they're both important for your health. Whole-food carbs supply soluble fiber and resistant starch to help you feel full, feed gut bacteria, and promote balanced estrogen metabolism, whilst fat delivers vital fat-soluble minerals and critical fatty acids.

Neither fat nor carbohydrates are intrinsically unhealthy. The issue is highly processed food.

Avoid eating ultra-processed foods.

The term "ultra-processed" refers to "formulations of food substances frequently modified by chemical processes and then assembled into ready-to-consume hyper-palatable food and drink products using flavors, colors, emulsifiers, and... other cosmetic additives." Almost all types of junk food, including chips, prepared sweets, fast food, and soft drinks, are ultra-processed. As you might expect, they are linked to a variety of negative health effects, including insulin resistance, heart disease, and fatty liver. Ultra-processed foods are devoid of the nutrients and fiber that your microbiome requires. In addition, they frequently contain harmful food additives, high-dose fructose, and processed vegetable oils.

Processed vegetable oils include oils such as soy, corn, canola, and cottonseed oil and can include one or both 1) trans fat, and 2) a high dose of omega-6 fatty acids. Trans fat is an industrially generated oil that's utilized by producers to make food crispy and extend shelf-life. It's commonly found in baked goods, microwave popcorn, and takeaway foods and is so bad for your heart that it's banned in some countries, When ingested as part of whole foods such as nuts, seeds, and brown rice, omega-6 fatty acids are not as harmful as trans fat and are useful and necessary. Omega-6 fatty acids are only a concern in big quantities when obtained from processed vegetable oil and junk food. High-dose omega-6 fatty acids can increase inflammation and fatty liver by competing with beneficial omega-3 fatty acids.

Although officially a vegetable oil, olive oil does not include omega-6 fatty acids and instead contains healthy monounsaturated fatty acids. Choose a high-quality brand of olive oil, as some have been combined with other vegetable oils.

Phytonutrients and vegetables

Vegetables are healthful because they include essential elements including vitamin C, folate, and magnesium. They also give fiber to assist satiety and nourish the gut bacteria, as well as a fantastic mix of anti-inflammatory phytonutrients.

Phytonutrients are plant compounds that exist naturally. They are known by names such as polyphenols, flavonoids, lutein, and resveratrol, and many have been studied for their anti-cancer and anti-inflammatory properties. Phytonutrients function by inhibiting pro-inflammatory genes and activating anti-inflammatory and anti-aging genes. Sulforaphane, found in cruciferous vegetables, is one of my favorite phytonutrients. It triggers the Nrf2 chemical pathway, which activates hundreds of detoxifying, anti-inflammatory, and antioxidant genes. Sulforaphane can be found in broccoli, cauliflower, kale, brussels sprouts, cabbage, bok choy, collard greens, and broccoli sprouts, as well as a few non-cruciferous vegetables like leeks.

Phytonutrients are best derived from vegetables and fruit, although they can also be supplemented.

Plant estrogens (phytoestrogens)

Phytoestrogens are a type of phytonutrient found naturally in almost all plant meals. Isoflavones from soy and lignans from seeds, whole grains, legumes, fruits, and vegetables are the two major classes. Phytoestrogens are so-called because they interact with estrogen receptors but are not estrogen. They bind to estrogen receptors so weakly that they effectively inhibit estradiol and are thus better classified as anti-estrogens. When estrogen levels are high during perimenopause, phytoestrogens have a favorable anti-estrogen impact and can help to lessen periods and promote healthy estrogen metabolism. Phytoestrogens derived from food may even aid in the prevention of hormone-sensitive tumors.

When estrogen levels are low during menopause, phytoestrogens can have a moderate pro-estrogen impact, prompting an extensive investigation into the use of phytoestrogen supplements such as soy as an alternative to hormone therapy. Unfortunately, most studies have found no conclusive evidence that phytoestrogen supplements can ease menopausal symptoms or lower the risk of osteoporosis. They can, however, boost the level of the testosterone-binding protein SHBG, which helps alleviate symptoms associated with testosterone dominance such as weight gain, hair loss, and facial hair.

Your ideal diet

There is no such thing as an 'optimal diet' that works for everyone. Instead, you have your best diet, which may or may not have a name. In its most basic form, your greatest diet is one that provides all of the important nutrients, including amino acids, while also making you feel good. It is a diet that is minimal in ultra-processed foods and so does not produce inflammation or insulin resistance. If you are prone to mast cell or histamine reactions, your optimal diet may also be low in cow's dairy or other histamine-producing foods.

Be content

Plan your day around big, hearty meals that include plenty of protein and perhaps a starch. You will feel content and able to maintain this style of eating if you give your body what it requires. You will also be less prone to snacking.

Snacks should be avoided.

There should be no reason to eat between meals unless you're fueling post-workout or intentionally aiming to acquire weight. Snacking regularly, especially on ultra-processed foods, can raise insulin levels, cause inflammation, and stress the digestive and immunological systems. Evening snacking is especially damaging and the polar opposite of healthy overnight fast.

However, if you're anxious or haven't had enough sleep, you may feel hungry and need to snack, which is fine. And if you're having trouble meeting your protein requirements, treat yourself to a high-protein snack in the afternoon, such as nuts or boiled eggs.

Eat with adaptability and joy.

Unless you have a sensitivity, such as severe gluten sensitivity, you can be flexible and enjoy a range of foods without concern about straying from your new diet. Eating should not be a stressful experience.

Don't forget the water.

Many facets of health, including brain function and cognition, benefit from staying hydrated. Choose between plain water and sparkling, carbonated water. Black coffee or tea is OK, but no juice or other liquid calories are permitted.

Chapter 6

MHT (menopausal hormone treatment)

Menopausal hormone therapy (MHT) or simply hormone therapy is the new nomenclature for what was previously known as hormonal replacement therapy (HRT). The name was altered to distinguish it from hormone replacement therapy for endocrine problems such as growth hormone insufficiency, and 'hormone therapy' is a better phrase because menopause's reduced estrogen is natural, not a deficiency.

Taking hormones with menopause has been and continues to be contentious, with the pendulum swinging back and forth between enthusiasm and fear, and recently, back to great enthusiasm. As evidenced by the patient stories thus far, many of my patients choose hormone therapy, and I fully support them in that decision. At the same time, some of my patients decide they don't need it, and I agree with them. As we'll see, the only time estrogen and progesterone medication are genuinely necessary is to prevent the long-term health hazards associated with premature or medically induced menopause.

Let us begin by recognizing three seemingly contradictory facts that are all true at the same time:
Menopause's reduced estrogen levels are a natural state, not a shortage. As a result, there should be nothing intrinsically disease-promoting or health-promoting about decreased estrogen or additional estrogen.

Hormone therapy, including estrogen therapy, helps alleviate menopausal symptoms such as hot flashes, mood swings, and insomnia. As a result, it's something to think about, perhaps while you're waiting for natural remedies to work. Remember that hormone therapy does not have to include estrogen; it can also include taking progesterone on its own, as we'll see in this chapter and throughout the book. It could also mean only using vaginal estrogen, which is quite safe and can save your life.

Estrogen and progesterone therapy may lessen the risk of osteoporosis, as well as the risk of heart disease and dementia, though this is debatable. In the context of our current food environment, estrogen may largely operate by reducing the natural change to insulin resistance that comes with menopause. You may be able to lessen your body's requirement for estrogen therapy by using other techniques for treating insulin resistance.

In this chapter, we'll go through the many types of hormone therapy. We'll next go over progesterone for perimenopause and estrogen for menopause before moving on to troubleshooting, where we'll go over side effects and other challenging situations.

Hormone replacement treatment (HRT) comes in a variety of forms.

They can: include various hormones such as estrogen, progestogen, or both (a specialist doctor may occasionally give testosterone) be taken or administered in a variety of methods, including tablets, patches, gel, spray, vaginal rings, pessaries, or cream

be taken or employed at different times
procedures might be cyclical (sequential) or continuous

The optimum sort of HRT for you is determined by a variety of criteria, including whether you've had a hysterectomy, your stage of menopause, and your personal preferences.

If you're thinking about using HRT, consult with your doctor about the best alternatives for you.

Hormone replacement therapy

HRT replenishes the hormones that your body generates less of as you age. Menopause occurs when your periods cease due to decreased hormone levels. It typically affects women between the ages of 45 and 55, but it can occur at any age. Anyone who has a period is affected.

These hormones are mostly estrogen and progestogen, and they are necessary for everything from menstruation, ovulation, and pregnancy to bone health.

Although testosterone is not officially approved for the treatment of menopausal symptoms, a specialist doctor can prescribe it.
HRT with and without estrogen
HRT entails taking both estrogen and progestogen (combined HRT) or only estrogen (estrogen-only HRT).
If you've recently had a hysterectomy,
If you had your womb removed during a hysterectomy, estrogen-only HRT is indicated.

If you have not already had a hysterectomy,

If your womb is still intact, you will need to take both estrogen and progestogen. Taking both helps to reduce the chance of womb cancer.

Estrogen can be obtained in the form of tablets, patches, sprays, or gels. Your progestogen can be obtained by the use of pills or an intrauterine device (IUS) such as the Mirena coil. Using two different forms of hormone will supply you with the combined HRT you require.

You can also consume or use a hormone replacement therapy (HRT) that already contains both estrogen and progestogen.

HRT can be taken in several various ways. Each has advantages and disadvantages, and you may need to experiment with numerous brands and methods of taking HRT to discover the one that works best for you. Consult your primary care physician first.

HRT is typically required for 2 to 5 years, though it can be longer in some circumstances. Learn more about when to use HRT.

Tablets

Tablets are one of the most used kinds of HRT. You typically take these once per day. There are estrogen-only and combination HRT options available as tablets.

Advantages

Taking tablets once a day may be the most convenient approach to receiving therapy.

Disadvantages

Some HRT dangers, such as blood clots, are greater with tablets than with patches, gel, or spray (but the overall risk remains low). Learn more about the advantages and disadvantages of HRT.

Skin patches are another popular method of administering HRT. They function by adhering to the skin on your lower body and gradually releasing small amounts of hormones into your body.

Patches are typically changed every several days, but each brand is unique. Skin patches are available for both estrogen-only and combination HRT.

Advantages

If you have difficulties swallowing tablets or are prone to forgetting to take them, patches may be a better option than tablets.

Patches can also help you avoid some of the negative side effects of HRT, such as indigestion, and, unlike tablets, they do not increase your risk of blood clots.

Disadvantages

Skin patches may not always adhere well, especially if your skin is moisturized. Patches can also cause skin redness or irritation, as well as leave a mark.

To avoid marks, apply the patch to dry, non-moisturized skin or peel it off slowly.

Estrogen cream

Estrogen gel is a growingly popular type of HRT. You apply it once a day by smoothing it onto your skin. Oestrogen is gradually being absorbed into the body.

You must use this gel in conjunction with a progestogen if you have not had a hysterectomy.

Advantages

If you are unable to swallow tablets, gel, like skin patches, can be a viable alternative. The use of gel does not raise the risk of blood clots.

Disadvantages

It can take up to 5 minutes for the gel to dry on the skin, so you may have to wait before doing anything else.

Spray Oestrogen-only HRT is also available as a spray that you use once a day. You apply it by spraying one to three times onto the inner side of your arm or inner thigh. You must use this spray in conjunction with a progestogen if you have not had a hysterectomy.

Advantages

If you can't take tablets, this is a good alternative.

The spray does not affect your risk of blood clots.

Disadvantages

Although you can get dressed in 2 minutes after using the spray, you must wait 1 hour before bathing or showering.

Mirena coil, or intrauterine system (IUS).

If you have a womb and are taking or using estrogen tablets, patches, gel, or spray, the Mirena coil, an intrauterine system (IUS), maybe a viable option for providing you with the progestogen you require.

The Mirena coil is implanted in your womb and gradually releases a progestogen (levonorgestrel) into your body.

The Mirena coil can also be used to prevent pregnancy and to manage heavy periods.

Advantages

The Mirena coil can be worn for up to 5 years and serves as contraception.

It may be an excellent alternative if you do not want to take or use a medication every day or if you have problems with other types of progestogen.

Disadvantages

Abdominal pain and bleeding can be caused by implants such as the Mirena coil. Learn more about the risks of using an IUS.

ovarian estrogen

Low-dose estrogen is also available as a cream, gel, vaginal tablet, pessary, or vaginal ring. This can help with menopausal symptoms such vaginal dryness, burning, or pain during sex.

Advantages

Vaginal estrogen has none of the hazards associated with HRT and does not increase your risk of breast cancer. Even if you still have a womb, you can use it without taking progestogen.

Disadvantages

This type of HRT will not assist with other menopausal symptoms including hot flashes, mood swings, or insomnia. Testosterone

Menopause, like estrogen and progestogen, induces a drop in testosterone levels, however, this happens more gradually. This can make you sleepy, impair your mood, and produce a decreased libido (sexual drive). It can also have an impact on bone health.

Although testosterone is not officially approved for the treatment of menopausal symptoms, a specialist doctor may be able to prescribe it for you. This is normally only indicated if you are postmenopausal, have poor sex drive, and HRT has not helped.

More research is needed to determine whether testosterone can help with additional menopausal symptoms. Testosterone gel is available.

Acne, undesired hair growth, and weight gain are possible side effects of testosterone use, but they are uncommon.

Others who come into regular touch with testosterone gel may also experience adverse effects. Wash your hands after using it and cover the area with garments to avoid this.

If you believe you could benefit from testosterone therapy, consult your doctor.

Tibolone

Tibolone (Livial) is a prescription medication that works similarly to a combination HRT (estrogen and progestogen), but it also has a testosterone impact. You take it once a day as a pill.

It can help ease symptoms including hot flashes and depression, but some studies suggest it may not be as effective as combined HRT.

It is only appropriate if your last period was more than a year ago (post-menopause).

Routines for HRT treatment

The method you take HRT depends on a variety of factors, including whether you've had a hysterectomy, whether you're in the early stages of menopause and still have periods (perimenopause), or whether you haven't had a period in over a year (post-menopause).

You'll take estrogen-only HRT every day if you've had a hysterectomy.

If you require both estrogen and progestogen, your HRT regimen will differ depending on whether you are in the early stages of menopause and still have periods (perimenopause) or have not had a period for a year or longer (post-menopause).

HRT in a sequential combination

If you experience menopause symptoms but are still having periods, it is typically advised that you take sequential (cyclical) combined HRT. Both pills and patches are available.

There are two kinds:
monthly HRT if you have regular periods - you take estrogen daily and progestogen for the last 10 to 14 days of your menstrual cycle each month.

3-monthly HRT if you have irregular periods - you take estrogen daily and progestogen for about 10 to 14 days every three months.

Every progestogen cycle should be followed by a period. Speak with your doctor if there is no bleeding during these times. Your doctor might advise switching to continuous combined HRT post-menopause if you began sequential HRT during perimenopause.

Chapter 7

Difficulties with the body, including allergies, thyroid illness, weight gain, and aches and pains

This chapter discusses physical symptoms, such as weight gain, aches and pains, perimenopausal allergies, and the well-known triple threat of thyroid disease, perimenopause, and insulin resistance.

Take a moment to ponder why your body must go through so many changes during perimenopause before we discuss all the symptoms and how to cure them. Your body adapted to a consistent supply of progesterone and estrogen during your reproductive years, especially your immune system and metabolism. Your immune system enjoys the calming and regulating effects of progesterone, so when progesterone levels drop, autoimmune diseases like thyroid illness, which we'll discuss, can take over. Similar to how your metabolism enjoyed estrogen's insulin-sensitizing benefits, decreasing estrogen can result in a change from insulin sensitivity to insulin resistance. It is impossible to emphasize the significance of insulin resistance for your waistline as well as your long-term risk of dementia, heart disease, and osteoporosis.

reducing belly fat and reversing insulin resistance

insulin resistance treatment conventional

The typical recommendation for treating insulin resistance is to cut calories, which is based on the incorrect theory that abdominal fat causes high insulin levels rather than the other way around. It's becoming more and more clear that insulin resistance causes abdominal weight gain, so just telling someone to lose weight is like putting the cart before the horse. As you'll see, I recognize the value of calories but advocate for increasing insulin sensitivity as a more specific approach.

Although not as successful as diet, exercise, and other treatments listed below, metformin is a reasonable option and helps to increase insulin sensitivity. Metformin can be used in conjunction with natural remedies, but not with the dietary supplement berberine for the reasons we'll go through. Consult your doctor about getting a blood test for vitamin B12 because metformin can lead to digestive issues and a lack of the vitamin.

Insulin resistance can also be prevented or reversed with the use of estrogen and progesterone treatment. Progesterone only becomes insulin-sensitizing in the presence of at least some estrogen, such as that produced by menopausal ovaries, whereas estradiol always causes insulin sensitivity.

Progesterone also works to lower testosterone, increase sleep, and raise thyroid hormone levels, all of which are factors in healthy fat loss.

Steer clear of testosterone and androgenic progestins as these drugs might exacerbate insulin resistance and lead to belly weight gain.

Reversing insulin resistance with diet and lifestyle

Movement

The best strategy to increase insulin sensitivity is to move more. It functions by increasing insulin sensitivity even when you are at rest and by enhancing glucose uptake into cells while you are exercising. Keep in mind that one of the most difficult aspects of menopause is sarcopenia, or decreasing muscular mass, which is the regrettable outcome of losing estrogen. Lunges, squats, planks, and resistance bands can be used to perform strength training in a gym or at home.

Protein

This crucial macronutrient helps you gain muscle and decreases hunger because it is so filling. Remember from Chapter 5 that you need more protein during menopause, particularly the amino acid leucine. An approximate calculation states that you require at least 20 grams of protein per meal, which is equal to a serving of 77 grams of red meat or 87 grams of chicken.

To maintain your circadian cycle and feel satisfied all day, try to eat a portion by 10 am. For breakfast, I suggest beef or eggs; if that seems overly filling, it may be because your stomach acid hasn't yet started to work.

Instead of forcing yourself to have breakfast at 6 a.m., try waiting until 10 a.m., when you start to feel hungry.

Alternate-day fasting

An easy strategy to increase insulin sensitivity is intermittent fasting, which involves alternating between periods of fasting and eating. You can develop the metabolic flexibility necessary for weight loss, a healthy brain, and relief from perimenopausal symptoms by restricting your food intake, even for a brief period. This is accomplished by training your mitochondria to burn ketones instead of glucose. The promotion of healthy gut peristalsis, the upregulation of anti-inflammatory cytokines, and the enhancement of brain-derived neurotrophic factor (BDNF) are additional advantages of fasting. As your body "eats itself", which sounds unpleasant but allows your cells the chance to remove and recycle damaged components and replace them with healthy new parts, intermittent fasting also encourages this beneficial process. Autophagy can lengthen life and lower the chances of dementia and cancer.

Alternate-day fasting, 5:2 intermittent fasting (reduced calories two days per week), daily time-restricted eating, or the eight-hour eating window, are some types of intermittent fasting. I prefer the latter.

Simply eat a typical supper around 6 p.m. that includes all three macronutrients—protein, fat, and at least some starch—to create an eight-hour eating window. Afterward, consume no calories until 10 a.m. the following morning. Eat nothing until 10 a.m. the following morning, when you should have a protein-rich lunch. You can change the times to sooner or later depending on your body clock, but keep in mind that the main objective is to fast overnight so that your body can enter the healthy condition of ketosis.

Exercise, fasting, and overnight ketosis induction are all acceptable and healthful methods. By breaking your fast with a "keto breakfast," which is a meal that is richer in protein and lower in carbohydrates, you can gradually prolong overnight ketosis. You might wish to consume some starch at some time (perhaps during dinner), which will naturally knock you out of ketosis momentarily but is good. Moving in and out of ketosis is easier and more peaceful than trying to stay there all the time. Additionally, eating carbohydrates with your evening meal can soothe your nervous system, feed your gut microbiota, and make you feel more satisfied.

Will you get hungry while you're fasting? First off, if you're already underweight or underfed, don't try intermittent fasting because you won't need it because you won't have insulin resistance. Second, if you're also trying to cut calories, avoid attempting intermittent fasting. The idea behind the eating window is to eat till you feel full during that period. Third, if you're used to nibbling in the evening, don't be afraid of hunger, especially the hunger you could have before bed. A small amount of hunger before night is beneficial when trying to repair insulin resistance.

Consider whether 1) you're eating enough during the day, especially enough protein, or 2) you need to start with a milder nine- or even ten-hour eating window if fasting causes you to snack or binge.

A low-carb or ketogenic diet

A ketogenic diet aims to maintain ketosis during the day rather than simply at night. You must consume fewer than 50 grams of carbohydrates per day and get the majority of your calories from fat to reach that goal. You'll still require enough protein as well as low-carb vegetables (like broccoli) for their advantageous fiber.

Is the keto diet beneficial? It can ease mental problems including memory loss and migraines. Although it is not the only method for doing so, it can also aid in the reversal of insulin resistance. The same improvement in insulin sensitivity can be made by increasing muscle mass, fasting intermittently, limiting carbohydrate intake, and avoiding fructose at high doses.

This leads us to a significant discussion regarding fructose and sugar.

cut back on concentrated sugar

The sugar found in soft drinks, fruit juice, desserts, sweetened yogurts, dried fruit, and morning cereals is referred described as "concentrated sugar" or high-dose fructose. These foods contain a lot of fructose, whether they are sweetened with high-fructose corn syrup (which contains 55% fructose), agave syrup (55% fructose), table sugar (which contains 50% fructose), honey (which contains 40% fructose) or dates (25% fructose).

Contrarily, low-dose fructose, the sugar found in fruit, is good for you because it 1) improves insulin sensitivity, particularly when combined with vigorous exercise, and 2) fruit contains healthy nutrients, fiber, and polyphenols to balance out any potential side effects of fructose.

What's wrong with fructose in excessive doses?

Fructose itself is not the issue; rather, it is the dosage. Fructose increases intestinal permeability, oxidative stress, inflammation, and fatty liver at high doses, which promotes insulin resistance. Because the majority of fructose is converted to innocuous glucose and organic acids before it can reach the liver or microbiota, fructose does not have the same detrimental consequences when consumed in small amounts.

Fruits in moderation don't contain enough fructose to enter the liver. But about midway through a can of soda or a big glass of orange juice, the small intestine probably starts to feel overloaded with sugar.

In conclusion, low-dose fructose is a good thing and a nutritious part of fruits and vegetables. As long as you have adequate insulin sensitivity and consistently exercise, moderate amounts of fructose from unprocessed desserts are safe. If you have insulin resistance, high-dose fructose from desserts—and particularly highly processed foods—can be detrimental.

Simply put, if you want to reverse insulin resistance, you must drastically restrict or eliminate sweet drinks and most dessert-type foods, particularly ultra-processed sweet foods. Whole fruit, dark chocolate, and treats made with non-fructose sweeteners like brown rice syrup, stevia, or xylitol are still acceptable.

I recognize that giving up sweet foods might be difficult and that it may necessitate some serious remodeling of your cupboard and shopping list. It may also include confronting the issue of sugar cravings.

How to Get Rid of Sugar Cravings

Yes, desires are unpleasant. They can also be conquered, which is well worth the effort because giving up sweets to cure insulin resistance means you will be less likely to experience cravings in the future (because insulin resistance creates cravings). I don't mean get used to desires or use willpower to resist cravings when I say overcome cravings. I mean be rid of cravings to the point that you no longer crave or miss sugar. Consider how nice it will feel to not think about sugar, with no effort involved.

The strategy is as follows:

Consume adequate protein, particularly with your morning meal, because protein suppresses hunger.

Consume filling meals that contain all three macronutrients: protein, carbohydrate, and fat. In other words, don't try to limit your overall calorie intake while trying to quit sugar.

Get enough sleep because it lowers sugar cravings.

Magnesium is beneficial to sleep and lowers cravings. Choose a start date when you are less stressed in your life.

For four weeks, abstain from all typical desserts and dessert-type items. (You can still eat entire fruit, dark chocolate, rice syrup, stevia, or xylitol.)

Know that acute desires will pass in twenty minutes.

Know that after seven days, all desires will be away.

You should be aware that by overcoming insulin resistance, you can help to prevent future cravings.

Recognize that you're fine. You are not a bad person simply because you crave or overindulge in sugar.

If you find it extremely difficult to stop eating sugar, you may be hooked. Symptoms include

seeking sugar even when you aren't hungry.

seeking sugar in response to bad feelings.

hiding your sugar consumption from loved ones.

Being angry or agitated at the prospect of giving up sugar; being unable to envision life without sugar.

Please don't feel bad or embarrassed. Sugar addiction, like any other, may be overcome with the correct help. Seek expert assistance from a psychologist who understands addiction.

I've worked with numerous patients who are addicted to sugar and have been disturbed by how they always blame themselves and their lack of control when, in reality, the root of the cravings could be quite different.

More approaches to reversing insulin resistance

We've been looking at techniques to overcome insulin resistance and have covered a lot of ground, including activity, protein, intermittent fasting, and giving up dessert. There are a few other factors to consider.

Maintaining a healthy circadian rhythm promotes insulin sensitivity. If you've been working night shifts, attempt to find a method to switch jobs.

Maintaining a healthy microbiome enhances insulin sensitivity, which may explain why regular antibiotics might cause weight gain. If you require regular antibiotics, your primary weight-loss plan may be to find a means to avoid recurrent infections. Finally, keeping a healthy thyroid hormone level is essential for insulin sensitivity. This contributes to the perfect storm of menopause, insulin resistance, and thyroid dysfunction, which we'll discuss
in more detail later.
Insulin resistance supplements and natural remedies.

Before we get into the supplements, please keep in mind that diet and lifestyle are more beneficial than supplements in overcoming insulin resistance. Prioritise protein, avoid treats and get your body moving. You can then select one or more of the supplements listed below, beginning with magnesium.

Magnesium

Magnesium is my first-line treatment for insulin resistance. A high-magnesium diet is associated with a decreased risk of insulin resistance, while a low-magnesium diet is associated with a higher risk of insulin resistance. Indeed, several experts have proposed magnesium insufficiency as one of the primary causes of insulin resistance.

Autoimmune thyroid disease

The thyroid is a butterfly-shaped gland in the front of your throat that produces thyroid hormone, which is required for energy and metabolism.

Thyroid disease is more frequent in women and increases with age, so if you're a woman over 40, you have a one in ten chance that your thyroid is malfunctioning. The most difficult aspect of thyroid disease is that it is often confused with perimenopause and vice versa.

Hot flashes, exhaustion, weight gain, body aches, joint pain, anxiety, depression, high cholesterol, digestive disturbances, heavy periods, irregular periods, hair loss, temperature intolerance, brain fog, and memory problems are all symptoms of hypothyroidism. Hot flushes, racing heart, hair loss, bodily aches, anxiety, insomnia, and weariness are all symptoms of an overactive thyroid (hyperthyroidism).

Consider the following perimenopausal symptoms: sleeplessness, brain fog, exhaustion, weight gain, immunological changes, hair loss, and heavy periods. As you can see, there is a lot of overlap between thyroid illness symptoms and perimenopause symptoms. This can make obtaining an accurate diagnosis challenging.

If the symptoms of thyroid illness and perimenopause weren't enough, there's also overlap with the signs of insulin resistance: weight gain, lethargy, high cholesterol, heavy periods, and androgen excess (facial hair).

Aside from symptom overlap, there is an actual interplay between the three illnesses in that:

Insulin resistance is increased by both perimenopause and thyroid illness.

Insulin resistance exacerbates perimenopausal and menopausal symptoms. The risk of autoimmune thyroid illness rises with menopause.

Perimenopause is so strongly linked to thyroid disease that some practitioners refer to it as thyropause, which is hypothyroidism accompanied by or triggered by a reduction in ovarian hormones, particularly progesterone.

Perimenopause causes thyroid illness in what way?

Loss of progesterone diminishes free or accessible thyroid hormone and can cause autoimmunity, which is at the root of most cases of under- and hyperactive thyroid. Perimenopause is so strongly linked to thyroid disease that some practitioners refer to it as thyropause, which is hypothyroidism accompanied by or triggered by a reduction in ovarian hormones, particularly progesterone.

Perimenopause causes thyroid illness in what way?

Loss of progesterone diminishes free or accessible thyroid hormone and can cause autoimmunity, which is at the root of most cases of under- and hyperactive thyroid.

Thyroid disease diagnosis

A blood test for thyroid-stimulating hormone (TSH), which is produced by the pituitary gland, is the standard test for thyroid illness. When your thyroid gland produces too much (or too little) thyroid hormone, it instructs your pituitary gland to produce less TSH. When your thyroid gland produces insufficient thyroid hormone, it signals your pituitary gland to produce more.

TSH and thyroid function have an inverse relationship, with high TSH indicating low thyroid hormone or hypothyroidism and low TSH indicating high thyroid hormone or hyperthyroidism. Hypothyroidism is the most frequent of the two conditions.

How high is a 'high' TSH level? This diagnostic criterion for hypothyroidism has generated some discussion. According to current criteria, your doctor cannot diagnose an underactive thyroid unless your TSH exceeds 4 mIU/L. In other words, you are regarded to have normal thyroid function until your TSH exceeds 4 mIU/L. The issue is that you may have functional hypothyroidism (insufficient thyroid hormone reaching your cells), yet your TSH is low because it is being suppressed artificially by inflammation, chronic stress, or drugs such as metformin. As a result, using TSH together with free T4 (the thyroid hormone thyroxine), observable symptoms, and thyroid antibodies is a superior way to detect hypothyroidism.

Thyroid illness treatment as it is currently practiced

Hyperthyroidism (excessive thyroid activity)

Hyperthyroidism (overactive thyroid) is treated with antithyroid medications such as propylthiouracil (PTU) or carbimazole. You may also be offered radioactive iodine therapy or surgical removal of the entire or a portion of your thyroid. The scope of this text does not allow for a comprehensive explanation of hyperthyroidism.

Hypothyroidism (low thyroid activity)

Thyroid hormone is the standard treatment and is usually administered in the form of levothyroxine, which is natural or body-identical thyroxine or T4 hormone.

Thyroxine must be transformed by your cells to triiodothyronine, which is an active T3 hormone, to be effective. Unfortunately, various impediments to that conversion exist, including chronic inflammation, stress, insulin resistance, and/or a common genetic variant of the deiodinase enzyme, which converts T4 to T3. If you have any of these problems, you may find that thyroxine (T4) merely works to get your TSH back into normal range, but not to make you feel better. Fatigue, cognitive fog, and depression are all symptoms of inadequate T4 to T3 conversion.

Combination therapy (thyroxine (T4) with triiodothyronine (T3)) is the remedy to poor T4 to T3 conversion. Combination medication is not a novel concept; until the 1970s, the normal thyroid prescription was 'thyroid extract,' which contained both T4 and T3. Thyroid extract, often known as desiccated thyroid, is a porcine (pig) or bovine (cow) thyroid gland extract that is still accessible today.

With the development of synthetic T4 medicine, guidelines shifted to T4-only treatment, which lasted for fifty years until recently, when the pendulum began to swing back to combination therapy. There is mounting evidence that, while some patients benefit from normal thyroxine (T4) therapy, others require both T4 and T3.

Diet and lifestyle recommendations for autoimmune thyroid disease

The following rules are for Hashimoto's thyroiditis and should be used in addition to (not instead of) thyroid hormone treatment.

Skip the gluten

Most Hashimoto's patients feel significantly better when they avoid gluten, and some study has even connected Hashimoto's to both celiac disease and non-celiac gluten sensitivity (NGCS). For instance, one study discovered that up to 15% of participants with Hashimoto's disease also had undiagnosed celiac disease and that these individuals were subsequently able to reverse their condition by adhering to a gluten-free diet. In a different study, up to 50% of Hashimoto's patients had positive HLA-DQ2 and HLA-DQ8 tests for celiac disease and displayed some degree of gluten-induced intestinal permeability.

Appropriate intestinal permeability

Gaps that grow between your intestinal cells, sometimes known as "leaky gut," allow proteins and other contaminants to induce or exacerbate autoimmune diseases by activating the immune system. One of three causes of autoimmune illness, along with genetic predisposition and an environmental trigger like a viral infection, is intestinal permeability.

Improve autoimmune thyroid disease, fibromyalgia, and other illnesses by reducing intestinal permeability. Determine and eliminate the primary cause of intestinal permeability, which may be a food intolerance such as gluten. SIBO, alcohol, and some drugs, such as stomach acid medicines, the oral contraceptive pill, and NSAID (non-steroidal anti-inflammatory drug) treatments, are additional potential causes.

Determine the cause of low stomach acid and treat it with an enzyme such as betaine HCL.

Determine and treat any deficits in zinc and preformed vitamin A, two minerals necessary for immunological and tissue health. Take into account a probiotic that treats IBS, such as Lactobacillus plantarum 299v.

Consult a physician

For instance, they might assist you in locating a chronic viral infection like the Epstein-Barr virus (EBV), which has been implicated as one of numerous potential causes of Hashimoto's disease. Supporting the immune system with zinc, selenium, and vitamin D are among the EBV treatments.

supplements for thyroid autoimmune illness

A few supplements for intestinal permeability and EBV have already been covered. Beyond those, selenium is the key dietary supplement for autoimmune thyroid illness.

Selenium

A vital vitamin for the thyroid and immune systems is selenium. In numerous autoimmune thyroid disease clinical trials, it was discovered to drastically lower thyroid antibodies in both Hashimoto's and Graves' illnesses.

Allergies

The start of allergy symptoms such as hay fever, eczema, hives, and asthma can be linked to perimenopause. Compared to other times in their lives, women are twice as likely to receive an asthma diagnosis during the perimenopause transition. Perimenopausal allergies result from the immune system's recalibrating, which we've talked about a few times. This includes a propensity for high histamine levels and mast cell activation.

The good news about perimenopausal allergies is that once you reach menopause, you'll probably outgrow them.

Salicylate sensitivity is another sort of "menopausal allergy," and if it develops, it usually does so five or so years after the last period. It results in headaches, flushing, and face edema.

Avoiding high-salicylate foods and beverages including tea and herbal remedies is the recommended course of treatment, along with glycine, which aids in the removal of salicylates.

Conventional treatment for allergies in perimenopause

The traditional conventional treatment is antihistamine medicine, which is a logical strategy, especially since the sedating variety of antihistamines can also promote sleep.

Progesterone alone itself has positive antihistamine properties. Contrarily, estrogen should be used with caution since it can exacerbate a histamine reaction.

Allergies related to perimenopause: diet and lifestyle

The primary treatment method for allergies is a low-histamine diet. perimenopausal allergies supplements

perimenopausal allergies supplements

vitamin B6

Perimenopausal allergy symptoms can be alleviated by vitamin B6.

It works by increasing the activity of the diamine oxidase (DAO) enzyme in the gut, which aids in the healthy clearance of histamine.

What else you should know: I normally recommend between 20 and 100 mg per day, divided into daily dosages (e.g., 30 mg twice a day). Be cautious, as a daily intake of more than 150 mg over an extended period can result in lasting nerve damage.

Quercetin

The bioflavonoid quercetin is a yellow pigment that has long been used to prevent hay fever and other allergy symptoms.

It acts by preventing histamine release by stabilizing the cell membranes of mast cells.

What else you should know: The therapeutic dose varies depending on the concentration of the medication, but standard formulae provide 300-600 mg taken twice a day. It is generally considered safe, with little adverse effects.

Pains and aches

Aching muscles and joints are a prevalent symptom of perimenopause and menopause, outranking hot flushes in certain studies. Back pain, osteoarthritis, migraines, fibromyalgia, and the throbbing of previous injuries, such as that broken toe from 10 years ago, are all perimenopausal pain symptoms. Although the specific process is unknown, the rise in pain feelings is commonly related to the loss of both progesterone and estrogen's helpful anti-inflammatory properties.

Perimenopausal insomnia may also play a role, because sleep deprivation, particularly deep sleep, can lower the pain threshold, increasing pain sensitivity.

If you're experiencing discomfort, consult your doctor to rule out other options, such as Hashimoto's thyroid illness, which is a major cause of body pain and plantar fasciitis, or foot pain.

Traditional perimenopausal body pain treatment

Although the evidence is primarily anecdotal at this point, estrogen + progesterone therapy can improve perimenopausal and menopausal bodily discomfort. According to one big study, women who use hormone therapy are less likely to develop knee osteoarthritis.

Progesterone can also aid because of its sleep-promoting and anti-inflammatory properties. In terms of conventional medication, I believe that hormone treatment is a better option than antidepressants or pain relievers.

Medication for pain alleviation. If you need pain medication, you'll need to talk with your doctor about which type is best for you. Low-dose amitriptyline, a tricyclic antidepressant, is the most commonly prescribed treatment for fibromyalgia. It is safe to take if necessary, however, it can induce weight gain. Be wary of the drugs gabapentin and pregabalin, which, despite expert warnings, have recently become some of the most often prescribed pain treatments in Australia. Weight gain, addiction, and despair are all possible side effects.

Finding the best pain treatment is dependent on determining the correct diagnosis. For example, if you have pain from Hashimoto's thyroid disease, If you have osteoarthritis, get medical attention.

Fibromyalgia diet and lifestyle

Correct intestinal permeability because both intestinal permeability and SIBO have been associated with fibromyalgia and may be the primary underlying cause. Refer to the section on Autoimmune thyroid illness in this chapter for more information on intestinal permeability.

Find ways to unwind. Select techniques from the Relax your Nervous System. Yoga, green exercise, and getting enough sleep are my top recommendations for fibromyalgia, which might be tougher said than done because insomnia is a symptom of fibromyalgia.

Make some mild movements.

Some exercise is useful because it builds muscle and promotes sleep. Excessive activity, on the other hand, can aggravate fibromyalgia pain and induce 'post-exertional malaise,' which feels like you've been hit by a truck for a few days. Start cautiously with brief bursts of walking or yoga, aiming to attain no more than 60% of your maximum heart rate. You can then expand from there.

Supplements that help with fibromyalgia

Magnesium

We've already talked about magnesium, so don't be surprised if we bring it up again. It's my first-line fibromyalgia treatment, and it's performed well in at least one scientific research.

It operates as follows: Magnesium promotes cellular energy production, enhances sleep quality, and protects the nervous system from glutamate's excitatory effects.

What more you should know: Dosing instructions can be found in earlier magnesium sections. If taking magnesium orally causes diarrhea, consider a magnesium gel or cream applied topically.

Chapter 8

Estrogen : Crazy heavy periods and breast pain

Perimenopause is a difficult phase for estrogen. Your final few years of menstruation may be characterized by higher estrogen levels than ever before, accompanied by the near-total absence of progesterone. The combination of excessive estrogen and little or no progesterone can result in irritable mood, heavy, painful periods, and breast pain.

The forties are perilous years for the uterus. referring to the generations of women who have had their uterus removed through hysterectomy, a procedure you may be offered if your periods become too painful.
There are a few things to bear in mind. To begin, understand that there are numerous modern alternatives to hysterectomy, such as the hormonal IUD and other surgeries.

Second, recognize that it is acceptable to seek traditional treatment.

That is true for any ailment, but it is especially true for perimenopausal heavy menstrual bleeding because you cannot be expected to endure such bleeding for an extended period. In a perfect world, you would have been able to begin natural treatment early in the process, before your periods became unbearably painful. If you did not have that opportunity, or if you are now suffering from severe adenomyosis or another source of significant bleeding, you may be forced to undergo some form of operation, which is not your fault. It's still worthwhile to attempt natural treatment since it can work, and even if it doesn't, it will almost certainly bring advantages to your mood or breasts.

Finally, seek another opinion. I've seen several patients who were informed by one gynecologist that a hysterectomy was their only option, only to find out that another gynecologist disagreed.

Heavy menstrual flow

Heavy menstrual bleeding is defined as shedding more than 80 mL of total menstrual fluid throughout your cycle, or a flow lasting more than seven days. Menorrhagia is the medical word for heavy menstrual bleeding.

What is the volume of 80 mL?

You may never have measured the real volume of your menstrual flow unless you use a menstrual cup. You can calculate it by calculating the quantity of menstruation products you must use. One wet standard pad or tampon, for example, holds 5 mL, or roughly one teaspoon, and a super tampon holds 10 mL. So 80 mL amounts to sixteen soaked standard tampons or eight fully saturated super-tampons spread out across your entire period. Simply modify the count if your menstruation product is not filled. A half-filled normal tampon, for example, equals around 2.5 mL.

In layman's words, you should change your pad or tampon no more than once every two hours during the day. And you shouldn't have to get up in the middle of the night to change a pad because your flow should decrease while you sleep.

If you're thinking to yourself, "Wait, what? You are not alone if you say, "I lose a lot more than that." It is possible to lose significantly more than 80 mL in a single period, especially during perimenopause, when bleeding can proceed to floods - and you can lose up to 500 mL (2 cups) in a single period. Yes, 500 mL rather than 80 mL. If you find yourself in this situation, read the rest of this section before consulting your doctor.

More than seven days of bleeding or bleeding between periods

Prolonged bleeding is an issue for two reasons: 1) it contributes to more menstrual fluid and iron loss, and 2) it's a pretty good indicator that something is amiss, such as adenomyosis, fibroids, uterine polyps, or anovulatory cycles, all of which we'll discuss below.

Menstrual clots are commonly associated with heavy flow because rapid flow outpaces your body's ability to produce natural anticoagulants. A few clots are normal, but if you encounter clots that are larger than a 20-cent piece (approximately 2.5 cm), consult your doctor.

a deficit in iron

One of the most serious issues with heavy flow, particularly heavy flow, is iron deficiency. Symptoms include weariness, shortness of breath, hair loss, and easy bruising.

Soaking through a pad or tampon in less than an hour, needing to double up the pad plus tampon, and waking up in the middle of the night to replace a pad are all symptoms that your period is heavy.

bleeding for more than seven days

 clots larger than a 20-cent piece

  restricting your activities owing to heavy flow

 symptoms of iron shortage such as weariness, hair loss, and shortness of breath.

Pain

The second most common perimenopausal symptom is pain, which can be 'normal' or severe,' but technically, I would say that no level of pain is normal.

Normal menstrual pain is regular menstrual pain that is not caused by an underlying disorder. It is also referred to as primary dysmenorrhea. An underlying medical issue, such as fibroids, endometriosis, or adenomyosis, causes severe period discomfort. Secondary dysmenorrhea is another name for it.

DYSMENORRHEA

The medical word for unpleasant menstruation is dysmenorrhea.

What is the difference between regular and severe pain? Normal period pain includes cramping in your lower pelvis or back the day before or on the first or second day of your period. Ibuprofen can ease pain and it does not interfere with your everyday activities. Normal period pain should go away with natural therapies; if it doesn't, the pain isn't normal; it's severe.

Severe period pain, on the other hand, is throbbing, burning, searing, stabbing, or shooting. It might linger for several days and occur during periods and sex. Ibuprofen cannot ease severe period pain, which can cause you to vomit and miss work.

Obtain a diagnosis

Perimenopause's heavy or painful periods are generally not something you can handle on your own. Consult your doctor for an evaluation if you haven't already. Even if you don't want the pill or hormonal IUD, it's a crucial first step. Why? Because comprehensive examination will allow you to examine all of your alternatives, including the option of progesterone capsules, which your doctor may not immediately give but can be useful for many forms of bleeding and pain.

When you visit your doctor, he or she will most likely prescribe blood tests, an ultrasound, and possibly a pelvic exam. One or more of the following possibilities must be evaluated:

Endometriosis, adenomyosis, and fibroids are all symptoms of primary dysmenorrhea.

Endometrial hyperplasia and uterine polyps are examples of anovulatory bleeds. thyroid condition

Von Willebrand disease is a coagulation or bleeding disorder.

These are the most common causes of discomfort or bleeding, and we'll go over them in detail later in this chapter. Pelvic floor dysfunction or bladder difficulties, as well as other disorders such as infection, adhesions, and pelvic congestion syndrome (PCS), which is the development of varicose veins in the pelvis, can all cause pain. Consult your doctor.

Just a quick note regarding anovulatory bleeding in case you're unfamiliar with the phrase. We discussed ovulatory vs anovulatory cycles, which is an important topic for this chapter. Anovulatory cycles occur when you produce estrogen but not progesterone, and they are by far the most likely cause of your heavy periods. Endometrial hyperplasia and uterine polyps can also be caused by anovulatory periods.

Anovulatory cycles are known by several names, which may help you communicate with your doctor: hormone imbalance, estrogen and progesterone imbalance, dysfunctional uterine bleeding, ovulatory dysfunction, unopposed estrogen breakthrough bleeding, and estrogen dominance.

Treatments for menstrual pain that are commonly used

Before we go into treatment recommendations for each problem, let's go over a few treatments that will come up repeatedly: the hormonal IUD, iron supplementation, progesterone treatment, and a dairy-free diet.

Hormonal IUD) We first encountered the hormonal IUD as a form of birth control. It also has the astonishing capacity to lower menstruation flow by 90% while improving pelvic pain.

You may thus find yourself in a scenario where the hormonal IUD is your best option, especially if your other option is surgery. As previously stated, the hormonal IUD differs from other methods of hormonal birth control in that it allows for natural ovulatory cycling and progesterone production. The progestin levonorgestrel (not progesterone) produced by the hormone IUD can induce ovarian cysts, hair loss, and mood disorders. Both the hormonal IUD and progesterone pills can be used to treat bleeding and other symptoms.

Supplemental iron

Heavy periods from any source can put you at risk of iron deficiency, which can lead to anemia, an underactive thyroid, hair loss, exhaustion, and a weakened immune system. Iron deficiency can make your periods heavier by reducing blood viscosity, creating a vicious cycle of heavy periods producing iron deficit causing heavy periods.

The first step is to undergo a blood test for iron stored in the body. The test is called serum ferritin, and a normal serum ferritin level is between 50 and 200 ng/mL.

The most prevalent cause of iron deficiency in women of reproductive age is heavy menstrual flow, although it is not the sole one. Other variables may need to be investigated by your doctor.

Heme iron from red meat is the finest source of iron, followed by poultry, eggs, and fish. Iron can also be obtained from legumes and leafy green vegetables, but it is non-heme iron, which is more difficult to absorb. If you have really heavy periods, you are unlikely to get enough iron from meals and will need to take a supplement or undergo an iron infusion. Take iron only if you are certain you require it, as too much can be dangerous.

Iron pills or capsules

The traditional iron supplement is an iron salt such as ferrous fumarate, which is inexpensive and high in dose but is poorly absorbed and can produce digestive side effects such as nausea, constipation, diarrhea, gas, or black stools. Iron chelate, which is iron linked to an amino acid such as glycine, is a gentler technique. It has a lesser dose, but it is more absorbable and has a lower risk of side effects.

Iron should be consumed with your largest meal and not with tea, coffee, or calcium supplements. You can improve absorption by taking vitamin C and iron every other day rather than every day.

Even with the greatest iron supplement, it can take several months to restore normal hemoglobin levels, and if you have particularly heavy periods, an infusion may be required.

Infusion of iron

An iron infusion is a substantial dosage of iron administered straight into a vein that can restore normal hemoglobin levels in just a few weeks. Although there are normally no side effects, some of my patients have reported temporary inflammatory signs such as fever. An iron injection administered into the buttock is another alternative, but it is uncomfortable and can stain, therefore I do not advocate it.

Progesterone

Progesterone tablets can be used to improve flow or alleviate pain. It's similar to taking progestin but without the adverse effects or breast cancer risks. Progesterone, on the other hand, has many negative effects on the breasts, mood, and sleep.

As we saw in the last chapter, progesterone may be overlooked by your doctor because it is now only licensed for menopausal hormone therapy and not for problems such as severe bleeding, endometriosis, or adenomyosis. Nonetheless, gynecologists I've spoken with agree that progesterone can be used for those circumstances, with a few caveats:

Because natural progesterone is milder than progestin, a higher dose is required to achieve the same period-lightening result.

Genuine progesterone may be insufficient for certain disorders, such as endometrial hyperplasia.

The cost of genuine progesterone is higher than a progestin.

Prometrium or Utrogestan costs roughly 50 cents per day, depending on the chemist.

Progesterone can be administered constantly (which may be required for adenomyosis or very excessive bleeding) or cyclically (two weeks on, two weeks off).

Normal Period pain.

Prostaglandins, which are hormone-like substances that have several physiological functions, including the constriction of blood vessels, induce primary dysmenorrhea. Period pain can also be caused by high histamine levels.

Perimenopausal period discomfort

You may have experienced period discomfort as a teen, only to have it subside to reappear during perimenopause. Period pain is frequent during both first and second puberty because there is less progesterone available to exercise it's helpful prostaglandin-lowering action.

Conventional treatment for menstrual cramps

The standard treatment for normal period pain is NSAID (nonsteroidal anti-inflammatory drug) medication such as ibuprofen (e.g. Nurofen), mefenamic acid, or naproxen. It's a realistic strategy, especially because it'll only be for a few days per month. It can also greatly reduce flow.

Hormonal birth control is another option, however, it should not be used for normal period discomfort because the following natural therapies work fast and easily.

Diet and lifestyle for menstrual cramps

To minimize prostaglandins, mast cell activation, and histamine, try a dairy-free diet.

Supplements for menstrual cramps

Zinc

Zinc is my preferred period pain supplement, and it worked well in a clinical experiment.

It acts by lowering prostaglandins and inflammation.

What more you should know: The typical dose is 30 milligrams taken immediately after eating.

Magnesium

Magnesium is another supplement to consider for many of the illnesses addressed in this book.

It acts by lowering prostaglandins and relaxing the uterus.

What more you should know: Magnesium can help with both prevention and acute period pain. To reduce prostaglandins, take magnesium throughout the month. To ease acute discomfort, you can also take a larger dose during your period. I advise taking 300 mg of magnesium glycinate.

Adenomyosis and endometriosis

Endometriosis is an inflammatory disorder in which tissue resembling the uterine lining (endometrial tissue) grows outside of the uterus. Endometriosis is most commonly associated with discomfort, but it can also cause bloating, digestive issues, bleeding between periods, and infertility. Endometriosis lesions are most commonly found around the uterus and ovaries, as well as on the fallopian tubes. Endometriosis on the ovaries is referred to as an endometrioma or chocolate cyst.

Adenomyosis is a disorder in which the uterine lining (endometrial tissue) is found within the uterine muscular wall. The most common symptom is heavy bleeding, although adenomyosis can also cause pain, missed periods, and infertility. Both endometriosis and adenomyosis can cause painful bladder symptoms such as interstitial cystitis (chronic bladder inflammation), which should resolve with the therapies listed above.

Endometriosis and adenomyosis are distinct illnesses, but I'm presenting them together because they usually coexist and respond similarly to treatment.

Perimenopause and menopause endometriosis and adenomyosis

You can acquire either ailment at any age, although endometriosis symptoms are more likely to appear in your teens or twenties. You may have already undergone one or more operations. You may not have noticed signs of adenomyosis until your late thirties or forties. It is possible to have both disorders, beginning with endometriosis and escalating to both endometriosis and adenomyosis.

Because both illnesses are caused by estrogen, symptoms may worsen during perimenopause but subsequently retreat or diminish throughout menopause. In practice, this is not often the case, and symptoms such as chronic pelvic discomfort, bladder pain, and painful intercourse can linger beyond menopause. Because endometriosis is not a uterine illness, discomfort might persist even if you don't have a uterus. If your discomfort persists beyond menopause, investigate whether you're being exposed to estrogen as a result of estrogen medication or insulin resistance, which causes elevated estrone.

Obtain a diagnosis

If you have endometriosis, it may have taken years to diagnose, but it should have been detected by now. Adenomyosis may still go undiscovered in you.

Endometriosis diagnosis

Laparoscopic surgery, often known as laparoscopy, is the current gold standard for diagnosis. It is a type of keyhole operation performed in the belly or pelvis utilizing small incisions and a camera.

Surgery may appear to be an excessive measure only to obtain a diagnosis, but it can also be an opportunity to remove lesions and thereby ameliorate the disease. Other diagnostic options include consulting (and being seen by) a skilled gynecologist or undergoing a new specialist ultrasonography method. There may even be a blood test one day.

Adenomyosis diagnosis

Adenomyosis can occasionally be visible on ultrasound, but not always, and it is frequently confused with fibroids. Magnetic resonance imaging (MRI), which your doctor may order, is a more accurate technique of diagnosis. Being in your forties, having children, and having had uterine surgery, such as a cesarean or fibroid excision, are all risk factors for adenomyosis.

Endometriosis with adenomyosis conventional treatment

Because there is no cure for endometriosis or adenomyosis, treatment can only relieve symptoms until menopause.

Endometriosis lesions, a small portion of adenomyosis, or the entire uterus can be surgically removed using laparoscopic surgery or keyhole surgery. The long-term success of surgery for endometriosis is dependent on the surgeon's expertise and training, as well as their ability to remove all lesions. Excision surgery, a type of surgery, is usually more successful.

Hormone suppression medications include the contraceptive pill, Depo-Provera, and Zoladex. They function by suppressing estrogen, which can be beneficial but is probably not as beneficial as you'd like.

Progestins such as dienogest (Visanne) and levonorgestrel (Mirena IUD) do not reduce estrogen but can help with symptoms. The hormonal IUD can also reduce menstrual flow by 90%, which can be lifesaving for women with adenomyosis

Progesterone (Prometrium or Utrogestan) functions similarly to progestin but with less adverse effects. Refer to earlier progesterone sections for more information, and keep in mind that adenomyosis may necessitate a high dose of 300 mg.

Because histamine and mast cell activation play a role in the pathophysiology of endometriosis, antihistamine therapy can help some women. Antihistamines can help alleviate discomfort and increase flow. Additional conventional adenomyosis treatments

The treatments listed below are just for adenomyosis, not endometriosis. Endometrial ablation is the removal of the uterine lining by one of various methods, including heat, electricity, or freezing. It's only an option if the adenomyosis hasn't spread too far into the uterine muscle, and even with the treatment, you may still need a hysterectomy.

Uterine artery embolization is a non-surgical method used to reduce adenomyosis by cutting off its blood supply. For adenomyosis, the operation entails a larger risk of problems than it does for fibroids, the condition for which it is more routinely employed. As with ablation, you may still need a hysterectomy.

Hysterectomy is the surgical removal of the complete uterus and can be performed abdominally or laparoscopically using morcellation, which involves breaking up the uterus into tiny pieces with a power morcellator, similar to a blender. Morcellation should be avoided if there is a risk of uterine cancer spreading. Hysterectomy is a drastic option, but it can be the best one, especially if you are still years away from menopause and hence years away from natural disease regression. If you keep your ovaries, removing your uterus will not put you into menopause.

Endometriosis and adenomyosis natural treatment

To comprehend the natural treatment for endometriosis and adenomyosis, we must first take a step back and consider the underlying cause of the illness, which is not estrogen. Oestrogen, for certain, plays a role because it is a significant driver of disorders once they exist. As a result, the standard medical strategy is to restrict estrogen. Unfortunately, restricting estrogen can have major consequences for mood and bone health, and it is not something that can be performed naturally. Instead, the best natural strategy is to concentrate on treating the immunological dysfunction that is at the root of both illnesses, particularly endometriosis. What exactly do I mean when I say immunological dysfunction? I mean that women with endometriosis and adenomyosis have an abnormal immune function, including changed amounts and behavior of immune cells (particularly mast cells), as well as a greater level of inflammatory cytokines and autoantibodies, which is comparable to what happens in autoimmune illness.

Endometriosis with adenomyosis diet and lifestyle

Be adequately nourished, particularly with zinc and preformed vitamin A, which are required for the proper functioning of both endometrial tissue and the immune system. Both minerals are deficient in a vegan diet, so supplement if necessary, and keep in mind that higher-dose vitamin A is not recommended during pregnancy.

Improve your intestinal permeability to protect your immune system from harmful microorganisms and the LPS toxin.

For at least three months,

Follow a gluten-free, A1-casein-free diet:

Gluten and casein can both drive (but not cause) immunological dysfunction and a gluten-free diet has been shown to considerably reduce endometriosis discomfort. Seek medical advice because you may need to consider additional dietary sensitivities, such as soy or eggs. A history of severe childhood eczema is a red indicator of probable egg sensitivity.

Because of the significance of histamine and mast cell activation in endometriosis and adenomyosis,

Try a low-histamine (dairy-free) diet:
A low-histamine diet may also be beneficial in the treatment of interstitial cystitis (bladder pain).

The metabolism of estrogen
Estrogen metabolism is a two-step process that involves the proper

elimination or detoxification of estrogen from the body.

The first step is conjugation, which involves the binding of chemicals such as glucuronic acid to estrogen in the liver. A sufficient amount of nutrients, such as folate, vitamin B6, vitamin B12, zinc, selenium, magnesium, and protein, is required for successful conjugation. It also necessitates that your liver be largely free of the endocrine-disrupting substances and alcohol's damaging effects. Alcohol boosts estrogen through impaired estrogen metabolism, and not in a favorable way.

Step two is conjugated estrogen elimination through the colon, which is more efficient if you have healthy gut bacteria. Unhealthy gut bacteria disrupt estrogen metabolism (and hence create estrogen excess) by producing beta-glucuronidase, an enzyme that de-conjugates or reactivates estrogen and causes it to be reabsorbed. The entire process is known as enterohepatic recirculation or "gut-liver recirculation."

How to Promote Healthy Oestrogen Metabolism

Understanding estrogen metabolism, particularly the role of gut bacteria, leads us to a few estrogen-lowering strategies:

Reduce or avoid alcohol.

Encourage healthy digestion and gut microbiota.

Consume phytoestrogens, which have an anti-estrogen impact by promoting healthy estrogen metabolism.

Consider taking iodine supplements, which can lower estrogen receptors.

Reduce your exposure to endocrine-disrupting substances

(EDCs), such as plastics and pesticides, which can impede estrogen metabolism.

Identify and correct insulin resistance to prevent the excessive synthesis of estrone that can occur in abdominal fat.

Endometriosis and adenomyosis supplements

Calcium-d-glucarate

The calcium salt of D-glucaric acid, which is generated from cruciferous vegetables, is calcium-d-glucarate. The glucarate, not the calcium, is the active ingredient.

It operates as follows: By blocking the bacterial enzyme beta-glucuronidase, it promotes proper estrogen metabolism.

What more you should know: The therapeutic dose ranges from 1000 to 1500 mg, and it is usually only beneficial if you have obvious indicators of estrogen excess, such as heavy flow or breast soreness. Because adenomyosis is frequently associated with an excess of estrogen, calcium-d-glucarate can be beneficial. It may be less effective for endometriosis, which is frequently associated with normal estrogen levels. One word of caution: calcium-d-glucarate can impair the effectiveness of certain drugs by hastening their metabolism and elimination from the body.

Zinc

Zinc is so critical for good immune function that zinc deficiency has been hypothesized as a cause of endometriosis immune dysfunction.

It operates as follows: It improves intestinal permeability, decreases inflammation, and alleviates pain.

What more you should know: The therapeutic dose is 30 milligrams taken immediately after eating. Refer to the previous zinc sections for more information.

Iodine

Iodine supplementation helps many of my endometriosis and adenomyosis patients, but it has not yet been studied for either ailment.

It operates as follows: It inhibits estrogen receptors and promotes healthy immunological function.

What more you should know: Too much iodine can injure your thyroid gland, so don't exceed 500 mcg (0.5 mg) per day unless advised by a doctor.

Curcumin or turmeric

Curcumin, the main ingredient in turmeric, has been studied as a potential treatment for a variety of inflammatory disorders, including endometriosis.

It operates as follows: It has anti-inflammatory and immune-regulating properties, and it inhibits aromatase, the enzyme that produces estrogen. It also suppresses angiogenesis, the formation of new blood vessels that feed endometriosis lesions, and soothes mast cells and histamine. Finally, curcumin can directly lighten menstrual flow by lowering prostaglandins.

What more you should know: Curcumin should be taken with food for optimal absorption, but not at the same time as your iron tablet because it can impede iron absorption. It is typically harmless, although it can aggravate salicylate sensitivity symptoms and is not safe if you have a coagulation or bleeding condition.

Fibroids

Uterine fibroids (also known as leiomyomas or myomas) are benign uterine muscle growths. They are, to some part, inherited, thus depending on your family history, you are likely to have at least one fibroid by the age of 50. There's also a chance it won't create symptoms and won't even be detected unless it's picked up by an ultrasound. As a result, most fibroids are incidental discoveries, meaning they are there but are not the source of your bleeding or pain. Only a small percentage of fibroids cause discomfort, excessive bleeding, or other symptoms such as a sense of fullness or urine frequency owing to pressure on the bladder.

Fibroids during the menopause

Because fibroids are estrogen-driven, they should diminish after menopause. If they don't, it's most likely due to a persistent issue with insulin resistance, which causes a high amount of estrone.

Traditional fibroids therapy

NSAIDs or hormonal birth control, such as a hormonal IUD, are usually the first measures in managing fibroids' pain and/or bleeding. The hormonal IUD, in particular, can be an excellent option.

Hormone suppression with medications like Depo-Provera or Zoladex helps decrease fibroids, but they also have negative effects such as osteoporosis and depression. Be cautious of the fibroid medicine ulipristal acetate (Esmya), which was recently withdrawn in the United Kingdom due to safety concerns.

Uterine ablation may be used to treat severe bleeding caused by certain fibroids.

Forced ultrasound surgery (FUS), which employs high-energy sound waves to ablate or eliminate a fibroid; myolysis, which uses heat or an electric current; and uterine artery embolization, which uses injected tiny particles to cut off the fibroid's blood supply. These treatments have a low risk of infection and discomfort but are often less risky than myomectomy or hysterectomy.

Myomectomy is the surgical removal of a fibroid that can be performed either abdominally or laparoscopically. It is effective, but fibroids can reappear.

The removal of the uterus is known as a hysterectomy.

Fibroid diet and lifestyle

Fibroids do not have a natural treatment. The best you can hope for is a slowing of growth until menopause when fibroids should gradually shrink in size.

Reverse insulin resistance because it is the source of fibroid growth.

Encourage proper estrogen metabolism since excess estrogen promotes fibroid growth. Because of the stimulating impact of estrogen, there is an increased risk of fibroids connected with alcohol, endocrine-disrupting substances such as phthalates, and the pill's powerful synthetic estrogens.

Fibroid supplementation

If you have insulin resistance, consider magnesium and inositol, and calcium-d-glucarate if you have signs of elevated estrogen. Consider iodine and vitamin D as well.

Iodine

Iodine is my favorite supplement for slowing and preventing fibroids from growing. Unfortunately, there hasn't been much research, except one study that linked fibroids to thyroid nodules and inferred iodine shortage as a likely underlying cause for both disorders.

It operates as follows: It inhibits estrogen receptors, lowering estrogen activation of uterine muscle.

What more you should know: Iodine is beneficial for any condition caused by estrogen, which includes endometriosis, adenomyosis, and breast pain.

Vitamin D3

Women with low vitamin D levels are substantially more likely to develop uterine fibroids, which may explain why fibroids are more common in women with darker complexion, who may have a more difficult time getting enough sunlight to produce adequate vitamin D.

It operates as follows: There is preliminary evidence that vitamin D reduces fibroid cell development.

What more you should know: The suggested dose ranges from 1000 to 3000 IU, and as we'll learn in the following chapter, vitamin D functions best when paired with vitamin K2. In the summer or if you reside in a tropical area, you probably don't need to supplement.

Breast discomfort

Finally, we come to breast pain, which is typically caused by the same high estrogen and low progesterone levels outlined in previous chapters. Breast pain can also be caused by excessive prolactin levels.

Obtain a diagnosis

If you experience breast pain or a lump, consult your doctor, who will most likely examine you and recommend you for an imaging investigation. You will be given a diagnosis based on this information, which might be fibrocystic breast disease (lumpy breasts) or mastalgia (breast discomfort).

Mastalgia can be cyclical, meaning it occurs before your period, or non-cyclical, meaning it occurs all the time and is frequently caused by anovulatory cycles. In either situation, the issue is excessive estrogen, which is highly stimulating to the breast tissue.

Progesterone, on the other hand, soothes breast tissue and can alleviate breast pain.

Conventional breast discomfort treatment

Choose a bra that is supportive, well-fitting, and does not have an underwire.

Pain relievers such as paracetamol or ibuprofen can be used on an as-needed (not daily) basis.

Medications that can induce breast pain, such as certain SSRI antidepressants, diuretics, the pill, and spironolactone (Aldactone), should be avoided (if feasible). Consult your doctor.

If progesterone is prescribed for something else, it can ease breast pain as a bonus. Although it would be safe, your doctor is unlikely to prescribe progesterone for the treatment of breast pain.

Breast pain diet and lifestyle

To help minimize histamine, which can aggravate breast pain, try a dairy-free or low-histamine diet.

Encourage healthy estrogen metabolism, including the reduction or avoidance of alcohol.

Phytoestrogens, such as those found in seeds and legumes, can have a beneficial anti-estrogen impact and promote balanced estrogen metabolism.

Breast discomfort supplements

Iodine

Iodine is the most effective treatment for breast pain. According to research, it can treat fibrocystic breast illness and may even lower the risk of developing breast cancer.

It operates as follows: Iodine helps to stabilize and suppress estrogen receptors, which are plentiful in breast tissue. Molecular iodine (I2), sold under the trademark Violet, is the best kind of iodine for breasts. I2 is absorbed more slowly into the thyroid and more quickly into the breasts than iodide, making it safer for the thyroid and better for breast pain.

A FINAL WORD

So, congrats on making it this far! If you're reading this, you're devoted to making your life the best it can be, regardless of your age.

We are all "work in progress," including myself.

I can't live as I used to in my twenties and thirties.

When I run, my knees and hips pain, so I walk more (and have more time to enjoy the landscape!).

I have greater lower back problems as a result of my excessive sitting, therefore I have to stretch more than ever before (I have discovered the joys of yoga!).

And because I need to keep an eye on my adrenals, I've started meditating for 20 minutes every morning (I never thought I could sit still for that long, but I've grown to appreciate my little bit of quiet!).

I know I won't feel fantastic if I don't do all of this. It's an obvious decision.

That's not to say I always get it properly! I'm not perfect; I try to follow the 80:20 rule: 80% healthy (mainly during the week) and 20% more relaxed (primarily on weekends!). It works for me and helps to keep me sane.

And if you're reading this believing you're fine, you might be one of the fortunate ones. I admire (and envy) you! However, the majority of women over the age of 40 will experience less-than-optimal energy levels, undesired weight (particularly around the middle), memory or concentration problems, and other symptoms that can indicate hormone imbalances. And if this describes you, I want you to know that you don't have to put up with it; there is help available!

If you want to feel well again, you only need to commit to either figuring it out yourself or seeking professional assistance. Hormone imbalances react excellently to a few dietary and lifestyle changes - you'd be surprised how quickly they improve.

We've all heard that it's difficult to break old habits.

You may leave this book knowing what you've just learned and go right back to following the newest trendy diet or workout program.

That is something I do not want to happen. My life's mission is to get every woman over 40 back to their best, because, as I've previously mentioned, it has such a large ripple impact on everyone around you that it's simply too big to ignore.

Changing your mindset after years of dieting to focus on your hormones instead is what works.

You must put yourself first at some time... And I want it to happen right now.

And, hey, if you can get your family to do the same, you'll be giving them the best gift you can.

I sincerely hope you will commit to prioritizing your health RIGHT NOW. After all, how many people's lives would be enhanced if you were at your peak? The benefits are unquestionably worthwhile. There is no other option for me.